Competency Management
in Long-Term Care

Skills for Validation and Assessment

Barbara A. Brunt, MA, MN, RN-BC, NE-BC
Kelly Smith Papa, RN, MSN

Barbara A. Brunt, MA, MN, RN-BC, NE-BC, Author

Kelly Smith Papa, RN, MSN, Author

Adrianne Avillion, DEd, RN, Co-author

Gwen A. Valois, MS, RN, BC, Co-author

Jane G. Alberico, MS, RN, CEN, Co-author

Barbara Acello, MS, RN, Reviewer

Adrienne Trivers, Managing Editor

Elizabeth Petersen, Executive Editor

Emily Sheahan, Group Publisher

Amanda Donaldson, Copyeditor

Amy Cohen, Proofreader

Matt Sharpe, Production Supervisor

Janell Lukac, Graphic Artist

Susan Darbyshire, Art Director

Jean St. Pierre, Director of Operations

Advice given is general. Readers should consult professional counsel for specific legal, ethical, or clinical questions. Arrangements can be made for quantity discounts. For more information, contact:

HCPro, Inc.

75 Sylvan Street, Suite A-101

Danvers, MA 01923

Telephone: 800/650-6787 or 781/639-1872

Fax: 781/639-2982

E-mail: *customerservice@hcpro.com*

Visit HCPro at: *www.hcpro.com* **and** *www.hcmarketplace.com*

Rev. 03/2012

50816

Contents

Figure List v

About the Authors vi

Contributing Authors vii

Preface viii

Introduction xi

Chapter 1: Why Is Competency Validation Required? 1

    Regulating Competence 3

Chapter 2: What Is Competency Validation? 7

    Competency-Based Education 9

    Defining Competencies 11

    Classifying Competencies by Domains and Levels 11

    Who Performs Competency Validation? 12

    Mandatory Training Versus Competencies 13

    Mapping Competencies for Orientation, Annual Assessments 14

    Methods for Validating Competencies 16

Chapter 3: Competency Validation in Job Descriptions and Performance Evaluations 19

    The Benefits 22

    Key Elements of a Competency-Based Job Description 22

Chapter 4: Train the Staff to Perform Competency Validation 27

    Developing a Competency Assessment Training Program 29

    Identifying Your Competency Assessors 32

    Keeping Your Validation System Consistent 33

    Incorporating Population-Specific Competencies 35

    Documentation and Recordkeeping 36

    Conclusion 37

Chapter 5: Keep Up with New Competencies 39

    Potential Categories for New Competencies 41

    Interpersonal Communication 42

    Guidelines for New Competency Development 43

    Best Practices for the Implementation of New Competencies 46

    Dimensions of Competencies 48

Chapter 6: Using Your Skills Checklists 51

Differences between Orientation Checklists and Skills Checklists 54

Skills Checklists for Annual Competency Assessment 55

The Competencies Analyzer 56

Chapter 7: Competencies 73

(See pp. 74–76 for a full listing of competencies.)

Figure List

Figure 2.1: Comparison of CBE and Traditional Education 10

Figure 3.1: Essential Functions 24

Figure 3.2: Rating Scale and Definitions 25

Figure 4.1: Successful Completion of Competency Assessment Training Form 34

Figure 5.1: New Competency Assessment Checklist 45

Figure 6.1: Skills Checklist Template 59

Figure 6.2: RN Competency-Based Orientation Checklist 60

Figure 6.3: CNA Competency-Based Orientation Checklist 65

Figure 6.4: Competencies Tracking Sheet 71

About the Authors

Barbara A. Brunt, MA, MN, RN-BC, NE-BC, is director of nursing education and staff development at Summa Health System in Akron, OH. Brunt has held a variety of staff development positions, including educator, coordinator, and director, for the past 30 years. She has presented on several topics, both locally and nationally, and has published numerous articles, chapters in books, and books. She served as a section editor for all three editions of the *Core Curriculum for Staff Development* published by the National Nursing Staff Development Organization (NNSDO) and coauthored *Nursing Professional Development: Nursing Review and Resource Manual,* a book published by the American Nurses Credentialing Center Institute for Credentialing Innovation. She was the author of *Competencies for Staff Educators: Tools to Evaluate and Enhance Nursing Professional Development,* published by HCPro, Inc., in Marblehead, MA.

Brunt holds a master's degree in community health education from Kent State University and a master's degree in nursing from the University of Dundee in Scotland. Her research has focused on competencies. She maintains certification in nursing professional development and as a nurse executive, and has been active in numerous professional associations. She is currently serving a two-year term as president of NNSDO and a term as second vice president of the Delta Omega chapter of Sigma Theta Tau International. She has received awards for excellence in writing, nursing research, leadership, and staff development.

Kelly Smith Papa, RN, MSN, is the director of education, research, and dementia care consulting at the Alzheimer's Resource Center of Connecticut. Smith Papa was a fellow in the 2007 Leadership AAHSA Academy and currently is the chair for the program's Shared Learning Alumni Committee. Her experiences in the field of aging services include being a director of nursing, clinical educator, nursing supervisor, and adjunct faculty member at the University of Hartford. She has presented at conferences and seminars for healthcare professionals on topics including creativity in staff development, person-centered care, culture change, dementia care specialists, making dining meaningful, and leadership development. She has authored multiple books and articles focused on the use of creativity in staff development and caring for people with dementia.

She was the author of the *Inservice Training Guide: Strategies for Effective Long-Term Care Staff Education* and *The CNA Training Solution,* both published by HCPro, Inc., in Marblehead, MA.

Contributing Authors

Adrianne E. Avillion, DEd, RN, is the owner of Avillion's Curriculum Design in York, PA. Avillion specializes in designing continuing education programs for healthcare professionals and freelance medical writers. She also offers consulting services in work redesign, quality improvement, and staff development.

Avillion has published extensively, including serving as editor of the first and second editions of *The Core Curriculum for Staff Development.* Her most recent publications include *Evidence-Based Staff Development: Strategies to Create, Measure, and Refine Your Program, A Practical Guide to Staff Development: Tools and Techniques for Effective Education,* and *Designing Nursing Orientation: Evidence-Based Strategies for Effective Programs,* all published by HCPro, Inc., and *Nurse Entrepreneurship: The Art of Running Your Own Business,* published by Creative Health Care Management in Minneapolis. She is also a frequent presenter at conferences and conventions devoted to the specialty of continuing education and staff development.

Gwen A. Valois, MS, RN, BC, is the director of education for CiNet Healthcare Learning. Valois has clinical expertise in pediatrics and has served for more than 25 years in various clinical educational and leadership roles.

Valois received her Bachelor of Science in Nursing from Texas Woman's University, her master's degree in HR management and development from National Louis University, and holds certification from the American Nurses Credentialing Center in nursing professional development.

Jane G. Alberico, MS, RN, CEN, has more than 30 years of nursing practice in healthcare. Alberico received her bachelor of science degree from the University of Kentucky and master's degree in health science instruction, with a minor in healthcare administration, from Texas Woman's University.

Alberico is a certified emergency nurse whose clinical expertise includes medical-surgical, home health, pain management, and emergency care. She has served in faculty and leadership roles in school and hospital settings. She is a national speaker for various topics and is currently the supervisor of clinical education at Medical City Dallas Hospital.

Preface

Before you use any methodology for validating and assessing the competency of your nurses to deliver safe resident care, it is essential that you have a system in place for verifying that your nurses are who they say they are prior to allowing them in your facility.

This might sound obvious, but stories of nurses faking credentials, hopping from job to job in various states, and harming residents are stark reminders that you must be diligent in verifying any nursing applicant's licensure, criminal background, education, and employment history.

Nurse-credentialing processes at some facilities may be inadequate. Nurses who have had action taken against them by another state nursing board, have a criminal history, or have incomplete education may slip by and end up working in direct contact with your residents, making those residents vulnerable and your facility liable. You should examine your organization's policies to make sure they protect your patients, and sufficiently screen applicants for dangerous nurses or imposters.

Credentialing nurses usually falls to the HR department in most facilities, and the administrative staff handles physician and advance-practice RN credentialing. For advice on credentialing nurses, HR administrators can consult their nursing directors and administrators, who most likely already have an established credentialing process in place.

The following are some steps you can take to verify nurses' credentials and to ensure your residents' safety and your facility's integrity.

Step 1: Gather Applicant Information

The employment application should be thorough and request the information needed to ensure patient safety in your facility. Ask for the following:

- The applicant's name and any other names he or she has used (e.g., a maiden name)

- Education, the degree obtained, and the name and location of the educational institution

- Professional licensure, the state in which the license was issued, the date issued, the license number, and the expiration date

- Disciplinary actions on the license

- Specialty certification

- Employment history

With many new nursing schools starting up, the organization needs to determine whether it requires nursing applicants to be graduates of an accredited school of nursing. New programs cannot apply for National League for Nursing Accreditation Commission accreditation until after their first class has graduated, which means that organizations that require graduation from an accredited school cannot hire any graduates of these programs.

That also requires that the accreditation status of all schools from which a potential applicant graduated must be verified prior to hire. Is licensure to practice as a nurse in that state sufficient? Whichever policy the organization decides to follow must be followed consistently and must be reflected in the job descriptions.

It is also important to determine whether the applicant has even been convicted of or pleaded guilty or no contest to the following:

- Criminal charges (other than speeding violations)

- Drug- or alcohol-related offenses

If either situation applies, ask the applicant to specify the charges and the dates on which they occurred. Finally, inquire whether he or she has ever been suspended, sanctioned, or otherwise restricted from participating in any private, federal, or state health insurance program (e.g., Medicare or Medicaid) or similar federal, state, or health agency.

Step 2: Verify the Applicant's Information

Verify, to the best of your ability, the information you obtained on the application. Even if you don't find anything, document each verification step to further reduce your facility's liability.

Some facilities hire a third party to verify this information, but most often the HR department performs this task. Either way, make sure a specific, established process is in place.

The best method of checking an applicant's qualifications is to use primary source verification, including education, licensure, and past employment. For the most accurate and up-to-date information, you should check the state board in every state that the applicant nurse has worked. Most state licensing boards post licensure information on their Web sites.

Many organizations require criminal background checks on all applicants, even if the state nursing board runs its own checks. Nurses may have committed a crime after receiving their licenses. In most states, the responsibility is on nurses to notify the state board if they are convicted of a crime, but they may or may not do so, which puts your facility at risk.

Another important part of the process is to check federal sanctions lists. If you hire a nurse who has been sanctioned by the Office of Inspector General or General Services Administration, you could be fined thousands of dollars. Reasons for sanctions include everything from defaulting on student loans to Medicare fraud.

The following are some other potential "red flags" to consider:

- **Gaps in job history:** HR professionals are well aware of this red flag, but be sure to ask about the gaps. Understand that there could be a perfectly good explanation, such as the birth of a child or a family emergency.

- **Moving from state to state:** When an applicant moves around a lot, his or her licensure information could be buried or lost. Therefore, be sure to check the status of the license in each state in which the applicant practiced.

- **Job hopping:** HR professionals are well aware of this pattern as well, and they will look twice at any applicant with evidence of it. But be sure to call each employer and verify that no disciplinary actions were taken against the applicant.

Step 3: Continually Verify the Employee's License After the Hire Date

Most facilities check nurses' licenses when they are up for renewal to make sure that they are current and active. However, it is crucial that you institute a process to verify licensure status more often as well.

Ensure that your policy spells out that it is the nurse's responsibility to report any disciplinary action taken against his or her license over the course of his or her employment. If your nurses do not report such action, they could be working on your unit with a suspended or inactive license without your knowledge. Many nursing boards post disciplinary actions against nurses in that state, which can be used as another method to ensure that all employees have a current license with no restriction.

Creating a new credential-verification process or updating your current process is a very important prerequisite to the competency assessment process.

Introduction

In this book, Chapter 1 outlines why competency validation is required, Chapter 2 defines competency validation, and Chapter 3 discusses including information on why competency validation should be a part of job descriptions and the performance-evaluation process. Chapter 4 focuses on the training needed for staff to perform competency validation, and Chapter 5 provides suggestions on keeping up with new competencies. How to use the skills checklists is described in Chapter 6. There are 100 competency validation skills sheets included in this book.

I hope you find the information helpful, whether you are developing a competency management program or refining ones you currently have in place.

CHAPTER 1

Why Is Competency Validation Required?

Why Is Competency Validation Required?

LEARNING OBJECTIVES
After reading this chapter, the participant should be able to: ✔ Design a competency plan to effectively assess employee competence

Regulating Competence

Does it seem as though regulatory survey teams visit you every day? Sometimes the survey is announced and sometimes it's a surprise, but the surveyors—regardless of whom they represent—are always concerned about "competency."

The definition of this word is in the eye of the beholder. For example, *Webster's New World College Dictionary* defines competent as "well qualified, capable, fit" (Agnes 2006). The American Nurses Association (ANA) defines competency as "an expected level of performance that results from an integration of knowledge, skills, abilities, and judgment" (ANA 2007). In healthcare, however, it's not so simple. Your staff members make decisions and carry out responsibilities and job duties that affect residents' lives. When the goal is to achieve positive outcomes—whether to cure or manage a chronic disease process or to allow someone to die a dignified death—will "sufficient ability" be good enough? Should competency apply only to clinical bedside nursing? Should an RN nurse manager have to meet the same competency requirements as a staff nurse? No, no, and no.

Evidence-based practice involves supporting your actions with research and data, and basing competencies in evidence is becoming the standard in competency validation. Researchers have identified best practices for patient care based on evidence, so staff members' competence should be assessed based on their provision of evidence-based care. By instituting evidence-based practice in your competency assessment, you ensure that the methods by which you are validating your staff members' skills are established and grounded in research.

Protecting the public

Regulatory agencies are rampant in the healthcare industry. Their purpose is to protect the public and to ensure a consistent standard of care for residents and families. Initially, there was only the Joint Commission on Accreditation of Hospitals (JCAH). Ernest Codman, MD proposed the standardization process for hospitals in 1910, and the American College of Surgeons developed the Minimum Standards for Hospitals in 1917 and officially transferred its program to the JCAH in 1952. A trickling of new agencies followed, and in 1964, the JCAH started charging for surveys. JCAH changed its name to the Joint Commission on Accreditation of Healthcare Organizations (JCAHO) in 1987 and as of January 2008 it is now known simply as The Joint Commission (The Joint Commission 2007).

The list of regulators today now looks like an alphabet soup. Political debates regarding the effectiveness of these agencies have multiplied in recent years. In July 2004, for example, Centers for Medicare & Medicaid Services (CMS) began to criticize the validity of Joint Commission accreditations.

However, since its inception, The Joint Commission has never had federal oversight (Knight 2004). In some cases, criteria for federally mandated CMS regulatory standards may exceed those of The Joint Commission.

For long-term care facilities, the agencies that guide and oversee care and, thus, require competency assessment may now include the following:

- The Joint Commission

- CMS

- State departments of health and human services

- State medical foundations

- ANA

- State Board of Nurse Examiners

- Health Quality Improvement Initiatives

- Occupational Safety & Health Administration

- Office of Inspector General

- Quality improvement organizations

- Agency for Healthcare Research and Quality

- The FDA

- Centers for Disease Control and Prevention

Add to this a list of your facility's competency assessment initiatives. Most of these initiatives revolve around the mission, vision, and value statements of the organization. Indicators may include:

- Resident and family satisfaction

- Physician satisfaction

- Employee health and satisfaction

- Fiscal responsibility

- Community involvement

- Risk management

- Continuous quality improvement

- Culture change initiatives

Those of us working in healthcare started our careers wanting to improve human life, and it is frustrating at times when it seems that the bureaucracy of regulatory mandates keeps growing. But the business of healthcare must consist of personnel who are caring and able to perform their jobs safely and correctly.

Remember that the provision of quality care and services depends on knowledgeable, competent healthcare providers. Every organization should have a competency plan in place to ensure that performance expectations based on job-specific position descriptions are consistently met.

You must design your competency plan with consideration given to:

- The mission, vision, and values of your organization

- The needs of residents and families served

- The extended community

- New services or technologies planned for future services

- Special needs required for particular healthcare situations

- Current standards of professional practice

- Applicable legal and regulatory agency requirements

- Organizational policies and procedures

In addition, the organization should foster learning on a continual basis. The administration and director of nursing should foster building a learning environment and hold the leadership team and staff accountable for expected outcomes. The entire organization must foster a work environment that helps employees discover what they need to learn for self-growth.

The return on this investment is a positive resident/family outcome, such as improved health, the ability to manage a chronic illness or dignified death, job satisfaction, reduced turnover, enhanced facility image, reduced risk of legal exposure, and improved surveys.

A consistent process for competency assessment is essential throughout the organization for all job classes, contract personnel, and, when indicated, affiliating schools. There must be a centralized, organized approach that moves seamlessly throughout the continuum of care and ensures the same standard or practice for all of the residents and families it serves. You might find yourself in a predicament if your main policies and procedures differ from other departments in your facility.

Generating tons of paperwork does not ensure competency in practice. Use the KISS method:

"Keep it simple, smarty." Although documenting that standards are being met is important, regulatory surveyors are moving away from looking at paper. The trend is to interview residents, staff members, physicians, vendors, and members of the leadership team to see evidence of compliance. And now more than ever, there are expectations to move beyond merely verifying whether nurses are competent. Thanks in part to advances in technology, nurses have been catapulted into more advanced and specialized care.

It is vital for you and your organization to be survey-ready every day. Ongoing performance must be measured and assessed. If individual members of your facility do not meet the standards you've established, individuals and the leadership team must develop a system for ongoing validation and assessment of personnel based on those standards. Remember: Competency assessment would be necessary even if it were not an accreditation standard.

It is worth framing this discussion on the expectations of regulatory agencies, because understanding their motivations and complying with their recommendations will result in a better understanding of what an effective competency assessment process should look like.

REFERENCES

1. Agnes, Michael (Ed). *Webster's New World College Dictionary.* Cleveland: Wiley Publishing, 2006.

2. ANA. *Code of Ethics for Nurses with Interpretive Statements.* Washington, DC: ANA, 2001.

3. ANA. *Position Statement on Competency.* Silver Spring, MD: ANA, 2007.

4. College of American Pathologists, *www.cap.org* (accessed November 25, 2007).

5. Knight, Tom. "JCAHO Certification—Dissecting an Institution." *The Nurses' Lounge* (September 2004): 26.

CHAPTER 2

What Is Competency Validation?

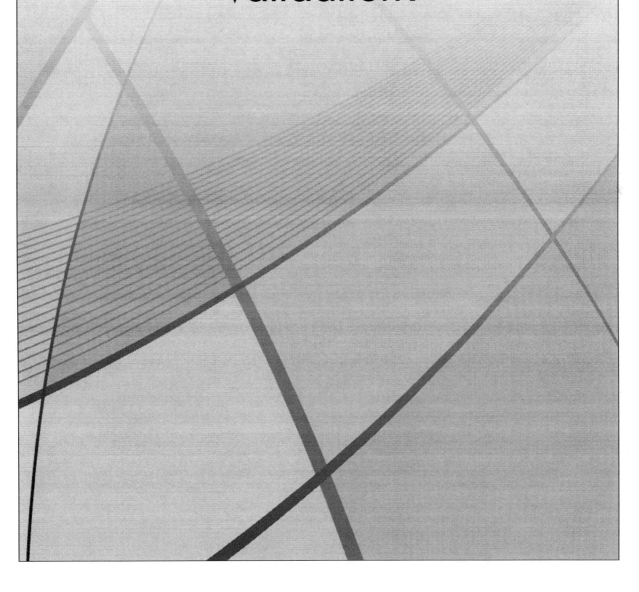

What Is Competency Validation?

Competency is an issue that affects nursing personnel in all practice settings. Increased pressure from multiple healthcare regulatory agencies and the public necessitates comprehensive evaluation of staff competency. The public demands that nurses demonstrate their competence. This chapter provides information on competency-based education (CBE), as well as on levels and domains of competency. Responsibility for competency validation and the difference between mandatory training and competencies are outlined. The chapter also describes methods for validating competence and options for mapping out or scheduling competencies.

Competency-Based Education

CBE is one approach commonly used to assess and validate competency. In many ways, CBE reflects a pragmatic concern for doing, not just knowing how to do it. Competency models began to evolve during the 1960s as an approach to teacher education; today, CBE models are a widely applied approach to validating competence. In CBE, the learners' self-direction allows educators to act as facilitators to promote learners' goals and is compatible with adults' developmental needs.

Barbara A. Brunt, MA, MN, RN-BC, NE-BC, identified that common characteristics of CBE include a learner-centered philosophy, real-life orientation, flexibility, clearly articulated standards, a focus on outcomes, and criterion-reference evaluation methods (Brunt 2007). Most CBE programs focus on outcomes rather than processes.

Generally, CBE programs focus on a specific role and setting and use criteria developed by expert practitioners. CBE emphasizes outcomes in terms of what individuals must know and be able to do and allows flexible pathways for achieving those outcomes. Figure 2.1 provides a comparison of CBE and traditional education.

A competency-based approach offers many benefits, such as:

- Having clear guidelines for everyone involved in the process

- Encouraging teamwork

- Enhancing skills and knowledge

- Increasing staff retention

- Reducing staff anxiety

- Improving nursing performance

- Ensuring compliance with the Joint Commission standard and Centers for Medicare & Medicaid Services' regulations that all staff members are competent to fulfill their assigned responsibilities

FIGURE 2.1

Comparison of CBE and Traditional Education

Characteristic	CBE programs (Learner-centered)	Traditional education (Teacher-centered)
Basis of instruction	Student outcomes (competencies)	Specific information to be covered
Pace of instruction	Learner sets own pace in meeting objectives	All proceed at pace determined by instructor
How proceed from task to task	Master one task before moving to another	Fixed amount of time on each module
Focus of instruction	Specific tasks included in role	Information that may or may not be part of role
Method of evaluation	Evaluated according to predetermined standards	Relate achievement of learner to other learners

 Competency Management in Long-Term Care

Defining Competencies

Confusion surrounding the competency movement is a result of the numerous definitions used to address this concept, and definitions vary widely. The definition used in this chapter is that competency is a broad statement describing an aspect of practice that must be developed and demonstrated, and competence is the achievement and integration of many competencies into practice, or the overall ability to perform. Competency is about what people can do. It is the integration of cognitive, affective, and psychomotor domains of practice. It involves both the ability to perform in a given context and the capacity to transfer knowledge and skills to new tasks and situations.

Classifying Competencies by Domains and Levels

Once an institution has a clear definition of competency, the next step is to classify competencies by domains and levels.

Domains of competency

Dorothy del Bueno, a recognized expert in nursing CBE, described three domains of competence—technical, interpersonal, and critical-thinking skills—that are often addressed in literature. Del Bueno developed a performance-based development system (PBDS) that focuses on these three aspects of practice.

The PBDS provides initial assessment data about a nurse's ability to perform and identifies learning needs. Clinical judgment skills are assessed through a series of videotaped resident scenarios in which the nurse must use critical thinking skills to identify the problem and outline the steps to be taken to solve that problem. This practice helps assess the nurse's ability to recognize and manage resident problems and give rationale for interventions taken.

For example, you can review a Kardex to see when a PRN was given and the desired outcome or to see whether the nurse is thinking critically about the use of PRNs when comparing them to the scheduled medications. Resident Kardexes and care plans also provide the opportunity to assess the nurse's ability to prioritize scheduled activities for residents, and event cards are used to assess the nurse's ability to determine the priority for unscheduled events. If a task is a must-do event, the nurse must identify the appropriate action to take.

Audiotapes of various nurse–physician or nurse–nurse interactions assess the nurse's ability to recognize ineffective interpersonal strategies and identify interventions that could achieve more desirable outcomes. Some technical skills are demonstrated in a classroom setting, whereas others are demonstrated on the care unit. After the nurse completes the assessment, the assigned clinical instructor completes a profile documenting the assessment, develops an action plan that summarizes the findings and identifies learning needs. The focus on technical skills, interpersonal skills, and critical-thinking skills is helpful, although the initial evaluation of competence for new hires may be too time-intensive.

Some roles may require competencies in other domains appropriate for those roles. For example, managers must demonstrate leadership competencies. In our increasingly diverse healthcare environment, it is important for staff members to demonstrate cultural competence when caring for residents of different backgrounds. Cultural competence encompasses not only racial diversity, but also diversity in age, culture, religious beliefs, sexual orientation, and other demographic factors. Cultural competence builds first on an awareness of one's own cultural perspective and then acknowledges the perspectives of another culture on the same issue.

Levels of competency

People function at various levels, and it is important to identify those differences in competencies. Pat Benner, a nurse theorist, differentiated five levels of skill acquisition in her novice-to-expert theory: novice, advanced beginner, competent, proficient, and expert. This book classifies competencies into three levels: beginner, intermediate, and expert.

Levels of performance are often differentiated by the ability to analyze and synthesize information. Beginners have limited exposure to the tasks expected of them and function at a basic level. With time and the development of expertise, they acquire more skills and can identify potential problems and act accordingly, at which point they reach the intermediate level. Experts have a wealth of knowledge to draw upon and frequently anticipate problems and plan strategies to avoid them.

A competency on performing a respiratory assessment would be a beginning competency for an RN, whereas initiating actions to prevent or minimize complications based on one's assessment data would be an intermediate competency, and appropriately responding to subtle changes in respiratory assessment data would be a more expert competency.

Who Performs Competency Validation?

After identifying expected competencies for each job classification, the next step is to determine who can validate competencies. This role will vary depending on the resources and types of personnel in the facility.

The American Nurses Association's (ANA) *Nursing: Scope and Standards of Practice* addresses the mandate that nurses must provide care competently and keep up with current nursing practice (ANA 2004). Individuals at all levels of the organization must assume personal responsibility to maintain their competence and ensure that they follow the system established by their organization to validate their competence.

Every organization has a responsibility to ensure that all staff members who provide resident care are educated appropriately and are competent to fulfill their job responsibilities and meet acceptable standards. To meet the requirements of The Joint Commission, CMS, state survey agencies, quality indicators, quality improvement organizations, and other accrediting bodies, organizations must also ensure the ongoing competence of employees (Joint Commission Resources 2008). To do this, they must establish a competency system and determine who can validate competence.

Various individuals or groups with documented expertise in an area can validate the competence of others. For example, a facility could determine that either RNs or licensed practical nurses (LPN) can validate nursing assistants' competency in taking vital signs. For lifting and transfer techniques,

Nurses or physical therapists could validate competency. For some skills, someone in one job category could validate the competence of another person in that same category. For example, an RN experienced in bladder scanning could validate the competence of a fellow RN's bladder scanning skills.

Organizations must clearly identify who can validate competencies and ensure that they have the appropriate education, experience, or expertise with that skill to perform the competency validation. Anyone who validates competence should be trained to do so (see Chapter 4) and should use an established competency checklist to ensure consistency with the evaluation process (see Chapter 6).

Mandatory Training Versus Competencies

There is often confusion between competencies and mandatory training required by regulatory agencies or institutional policy. Most facilities require that all staff members annually review a variety of safety topics, such as fire safety, dealing with emergency situations (e.g., cardiac arrests, choking, disasters, hazardous materials, and missing residents), and cultural diversity. Institutions have several ways to achieve this task. Some distribute self-learning packets (SLP) containing the essential information and require everyone to review that material annually. Some SLPs may require that the individual take a posttest, and others may require simply that the individual read the information. Facilities that have computer capabilities may require personnel to complete safety training programs online. Some may hold face-to-face sessions, which may include some hands-on practice

with the skill, for reviewing the information. The difference between mandatory training and competency validation is that the latter requires demonstration of the skill, whereas the former does not necessarily do so. To further clarify the difference, the following list outlines some of the common safety topics required by regulatory agencies:

- Cultural competence and ethical conduct

- Privacy and confidentiality issues (e.g., Health Insurance Portability and Accountability Act of 1996 requirements)

- Fire safety

- Disaster preparedness

- Emergency codes

- Electrical safety

- Infection control and bloodborne pathogens

- Institutional safety plan and resident safety

- Back safety

- Emergency response to various threats (e.g., bombs, resident/family violence)

- Caring for people with dementia

- Residents' rights

- Abuse prevention

Many organizations require that personnel maintain competence in basic life support or Heartsaver, which requires a staff member to complete appropriate courses as a healthcare provider, heartsaver, or advanced cardiac life-support provider.

The focus of competencies is on what the individual can do, not what he or she knows, and competencies must be measured in a simulated or clinical setting. One example of a competency that can be demonstrated without specific resident contact is blood-glucose testing. Any healthcare provider who tests blood sugar results must get an accurate reading, because treatment is based on those results.

Mapping Competencies for Orientation, Annual Assessments

You can determine which skills should be evaluated each year in a variety of ways. Selected competencies can be based on the needs of an individual unit, identified quality-improvement needs or problems, changes in resident population, care modalities, or new technologies. Summarized performance appraisal results could be used to indicate the particular competencies staff members need to develop further. Skills that are not used frequently but present high risk to the resident can also be validated. Most institutions require some safety training annually, as well as CPR courses; these can also be part of the competency process. Many organizations are working toward integrating their performance appraisal and competency management systems. We will discuss this further in Chapter 3.

Some facilities focus on skills that are high risk, low volume, or problem prone (Cooper 2002). For example:

- **High-risk activities** can cause serious (or deadly) damage to a resident or staff member if performed incorrectly. Look at high-risk activities closely. If they are performed every day, they are considered high volume.

High-volume activities do not necessarily need to be reviewed every year, although they should be part of your orientation program. The assumption is that you perform the activity so often that you know it well.

- **Low-volume skills** are not performed often within your department, but employees still need to know how to perform them well. These skills should be reviewed at least annually. If an activity is high risk and low volume, you should include it in your annual review.

- **Problem-prone skills** are the subject of unusual-occurrence reports or other error-reporting forms or quality-assurance data. These data should be reviewed regularly, because they are an excellent source of skill or knowledge deficits that become annual competencies. Near misses are also serious enough for a review.

Elizabeth Parsons and Mary Bona Capka suggested a model to determine how frequently skills should be assessed based on risk (Parsons and Bona Capka 1997). Although this may be more detailed than necessary for some organizations, it may be helpful to identify high-risk procedures. The following are key factors in their model:

- **Incident frequency.** This is determined by a rating scale that includes occurrence, quality improvement, and compliance data. Occurrence scores are ranked on a Likert-type scale (i.e., 5 = daily; 4 = once per week; 3 = once per month; 2 = once in six months; 1 = once per year or less; 0 = never). Incidents are defined as untoward incidents, equipment problems, staff noncompliance, or infection control data reported in the past 12 months. The more incidents, the higher the score.

- **Use/performance frequency.** This identifies the equipment use or competency performance. It uses the same Likert-type scale as the incident frequency scale, but with reversed scoring (i.e., 5 = once per year or less; 1 = daily). If procedures are performed infrequently, important steps may be inadvertently omitted. The more frequently the staff member performs the competency, the lower the score.

- **Resident/operator risk.** This scale scores each item according to the risk to the resident or operator if the competency is performed incorrectly. The highest score (i.e., 5 = operator or resident death) is assigned to competencies for which there is great risk to the resident or staff member, whereas the lowest score (i.e., 1 = barely any risk) is used if there is no significant risk to the resident or staff member.

- **Skill complexity.** This score captures the skill's complexity and is based on Benner's novice-to-expert model. Skills that the new graduate should be able to perform without supervision would rank lowest (1 or 2), whereas skills that require application of theoretical principles in creative and innovative ways score highest (9 or 10). In this manner, skills necessary to perform an identified competency factor into decisions made about the frequency of assessment.

The formula that Parsons and Bona Capka used captured all of these components, with risk being identified as the most crucial factor. Additional weight or value was given to the resident/operator risk score. Their formula appears in the box that follows. Scores range from 0 to 100.

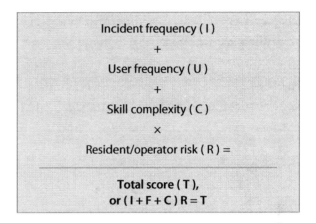

Incident frequency (I)
+
User frequency (U)
+
Skill complexity (C)
×
Resident/operator risk (R) =
_____
Total score (T),
or (I + F + C) R = T

For example, a skill such as providing immediate support for a cardiac arrest (e.g., CPR or advanced life support) would have a relatively high-risk score. The incident frequency would encompass the number of untoward events during codes in the past year (in this case, 1). User frequency would vary, but for most noncritical-care areas, it would be rated high (a rating of 5) because it is not routinely performed in those areas. Complexity would be rather high (a rating of 8) because a code is a complex care situation, and the risk would be high (a rating of 5) because inappropriate performance of the competency could lead to resident death. A potential score of 70 could be obtained using the formula given earlier: (1 + 5 + 8) 5 = 70.

Your method for mapping competencies to be validated needs to be flexible enough to allow for changes or modifications based on environmental factors. For example, a new piece of equipment might require the staff to demonstrate competency in using that equipment. The system would need to be flexible enough to include that as an additional competency in a timely manner for the affected staff members.

Methods for Validating Competencies

It is important to realize that there are numerous ways to validate competencies. One of the most common methods is the skills checklist, which is described in Chapter 6. However, there are many other ways that competence can be validated (Avillion, Brunt, and Ferrell 2007).

Posttests

Posttests are one method for documenting cognitive knowledge and are sometimes used as a method for documenting competence. However, when competency is defined as the overall ability to perform, many tests do not have a performance aspect. One way that tests can be used is to document basic knowledge so that participants don't have to take a course or program when they can show that they have the basic knowledge required in that course. Some tests may provide a written description, a videotape or audiotape, a live simulation, or printed or projected still pictures, and then present specific questions to which the test taker must respond. Del Bueno's PBDS uses this approach to validate competency.

Observations of daily work

Observations of daily work, such as rounds, care audits or medical record reviews, can be a means of validating competency. Specific interactions or skills can be directly observed as someone performs his or her work, and resident outcomes/documentation can be observed as well. This provides an opportunity for multiple observations and addresses one of the problems with checklists, which usually gather data from only one observation of a

task. When staff members know they are being observed, they have a tendency to go through all of the steps correctly when they might not normally do so. Observations of staff members caring for people with dementia can confirm that they understand the essentials of communication, approach, and validation techniques.

Case studies

Case studies are another means of validating competency. Individuals can describe how they would provide care for a particular resident or how they would deal with a particular scenario presented to them. These can also be used to address caring for challenging residents. After someone describes how he or she would take care of a resident who becomes aggressive, the assessor could ask that person what he or she would do to prevent aggressive behavior. The person's description of the skills he or she would consider and how he or she would alter the resident's care could be used to document the person's ability to care for residents with dementia.

Peer review/360° evaluation

Peer review, or a technique called "360° evaluation," is another method for validating competency. The 360° evaluation incorporates feedback from as many people who interact with a staff member as is feasible. For an RN, such people might include his or her manager, peers, LPNs, CNAs, and representatives of other disciplines. The use of different sources of information and different measures to evaluate competence increases validity.

Exemplars

Exemplars are narrative descriptions of practice. Individuals describe how they handled a particular situation; in essence, they write or tell a story about it. Their narrative allows the clinician to describe the step-by-step progression of the incident, as well as the feelings, thoughts, and conclusions from their reflection of the situation. These exemplars can be part of portfolios that provide concrete examples of competence in a particular area.

Simulated events

Simulated events, such as mock codes, can also be used to validate competency. For example, the instructor can use a mannequin and ask the participants to respond appropriately to a certain scenario. This provides an opportunity for practice and demonstration of skills in a nonthreatening environment. Another example is the use of volunteers as simulated residents for staff members to perform assessments or demonstrate various skills. Also available are various simulators that provide a realistic environment for demonstration of skills, but these can be costly. A disaster drill can be simulated to ensure that the staff will know how to act in a disaster emergency. For example, volunteers can act as residents who need to be transferred from one section of the facility to another due to water damage or fire.

Quality improvement monitors

Quality improvement monitors, if they reflect individual performance, are another method for validating competency. These are often related to quality-of-care issues such as falls, documentation, and facility-acquired infections. With the ongoing emphasis on performance improvement and quality, most facilities have a quality-improvement program and quality monitors in place. For example, a facility may document compliance with the new HIPAA security requirements by having individuals without name tags approach staff members and tell them that they work for IT services. They may ask the employees for their passwords to check the computer system or tell a secretary they are responding to a call about a computer problem and remove a piece of computer equipment from his or her manager's office. If the employee does not follow the established policy, feedback and follow-up are provided.

Scheduling and organizing the competencies

Once the competencies to be validated are determined, the organization needs to communicate them to all staff members and provide the tools necessary to validate those skills. This can be done in several ways. Access to the various checklists or methods to validate competencies should be available for all staff members to use during the validation process.

Some facilities may choose to have competency notebooks on each unit that include a tracking sheet of employees and a list of which competencies need validation for each role. Samples of skills checklists or other methods to validate competencies should also be included in the notebook. If a computer-tracking system is in place, this can be used to map individual- or role-specific competencies. Then the person who performs the validation could enter that information directly into the computer system.

Some facilities may choose to put the responsibility on individuals to make sure that they are validated on the required competencies annually. In this case, the individual is responsible for having the appropriate person validate the skill and would be responsible for ensuring that the appropriate documentation was completed. These data can then be used in the individual's performance appraisal.

Some institutions may schedule various competencies to be completed by everyone in a designated time frame (e.g., during the first quarter, two months before their annual performance appraisal, or at a scheduled skills fair). Others may allow competency validation to be done anytime during the year, as long as it is completed by a designated deadline. Whichever system the organization uses to ensure that competence is validated must be communicated to all staff members, and a mechanism needs to be put in place to ensure that the process is followed.

A final step in the competency validation process is to set up a mechanism for ongoing review and evaluation of the process. Specific questions to be included in an evaluation of a competence assessment system are provided in Chapter 6.

REFERENCES

1. American Nurses Association. *Nursing: Scope and Standards of Practice.* Washington, DC: ANA, 2004.

2. Avillion, Adrianne E., Brunt, Barbara A., and Ferrell, Mary Jane. *Nursing Professional Development Review and Resource Manual.* Silver Spring, MD: Institute for Credentialing Innovation, 2007.

3. Brunt, Barbara A. *Competencies for Staff Educators: Tools to Evaluate and Enhance Nursing Professional Development.* Marblehead, MA: HCPro, Inc., 2007.

4. Cooper, D. "The 'C' Word: Competency." *Staff Development Nursing Secrets.* Philadelphia: Hanley & Belfus, 2002.

5. Joint Commission Resources. *Comprehensive Accreditation Manual for Hospitals: The Official Handbook.* Oakbrook Terrace, IL: Joint Commission Resources, 2008.

6. Parsons, Elizabeth C., and Bona Capka, Mary. "Building a successful risk-based competency assessment model." *AORN Journal* 66(6) (1997): 1065–1071.

Competency Validation in Job Descriptions and Performance Evaluations

Competency Validation in Job Descriptions and Performance Evaluations

LEARNING OBJECTIVES

After reading this chapter, the participant should be able to:

✓ Recognize the benefits of incorporating competency assessment into job descriptions and performance evaluation tools

✓ Discuss the key elements required of performance-based job descriptions

New technology, legislation, and accreditation standards are changing the job responsibilities of those employed at your facility almost every day. In some cases, these forces may make it necessary for you to create entirely new job positions to keep pace and ensure safe, quality care. As a result, it is more difficult for administration to keep job descriptions current, create effective and realistic performance evaluations that are in sync with those job descriptions, and include these tools in a process for assessing initial and ongoing competencies.

In this chapter, we will provide further support for the underpinning theme throughout this book: manageability. That is, not only should you make your competency validation and assessment process compliant and effective, but you should also make it manageable. This chapter discusses the elements required to build competency-based job descriptions.

Competency-based (sometimes called performance-based) job descriptions state employee responsibilities in terms of practice standards, or how these responsibilities must be demonstrated, rather than simply listing duties and responsibilities. Competency-based job descriptions can double as performance evaluation tools.

Although these tools will take a good deal of time to develop, they will help your organization have a more streamlined system for developing performance criteria for your competency validation skill sheets, for assessing population-specific competencies, and for tying those assessments into timely performance evaluations. In this chapter, we will discuss:

- The benefits of incorporating competency assessment into your job descriptions and performance evaluation tools

- What the state department of public health, Centers for Medicare & Medicaid Services or The Joint Commission expect from long-term care

- The key elements required of performance-based job descriptions

- Practical tips for timely completion of performance evaluations

The Benefits

You can expect several benefits from incorporating competency assessment into its job descriptions and performance evaluations, including improved:

- **Efficiency.** As long as you are willing to put the time and effort into building competency-based HR tools, your reward will be a more streamlined, compliant competency assessment process. The performance criteria in your job descriptions can serve as the foundation for your competency validation tools (e.g., skill sheets) and performance evaluations.

- **Resident safety.** Defining employees' job responsibilities by widely accepted standards or scopes of practice and holding employees to them will help your organization ensure that resident care is delivered in the safest way possible.

- **Employee satisfaction.** Employees need validation from their managers or supervisors about their job performance. They need to know what expectations they have or have not met. Well-developed HR tools composed of measurable performance criteria will make it easier for employees to receive this type of validation.

Key Elements of a Competency-Based Job Description

What makes a job description competency- or performance-based?

The foundation for each employee's job description should be the position's qualifications, duties, and responsibilities. However, well-developed competency- or performance-based job descriptions at your facility must state employee responsibilities (i.e., essential functions and nonessential functions) in terms of expected practice standards—in other words, how the responsibilities must be demonstrated. Created by the department manager and understood by the HR department, these standards must have measurable, objective outcomes associated with them. The problem with many job descriptions is that they are written in a way that leads to subjective interpretations by supervisors.

Include an associated rating scale, which provides definitions that have been agreed upon across departments. This scale must be clear and easy to understand for everyone using it. Also include within job descriptions an area for a supervisor to document in narrative format how the employee met expectations.

Essential and nonessential functions

Essential functions are tasks, duties, and responsibilities that constitute the context of the job (i.e., the means of accomplishing the job's purpose and objectives). The essential functions should be measurable statements that cover the major components of the job for which the person will be held accountable. Figure 3.1 shows an example of two essential functions and their expected performance criteria.

Functions listed as nonessential aren't unimportant—they just are not critical for the performance of the job position. They should be listed as specifically as possible and include performance criteria.

Organizational competencies

Job descriptions should also include organizational competencies—those that are expected across all departments of the organization for every employee. This will often require you to incorporate competency-based performance standards in sections devoted to but not limited to:

- Service

- Teamwork

- Communication

- Respect for others

- Time and priority management

- Mandatory safety requirements

- Leadership competencies

Rating scale and definitions

The rating-scale portion of your job descriptions is extremely important. To develop a rating scale, consider:

- How many levels of ratings are required to differentiate performance

- How many standards can be identified, maintained, and discriminated in your performance appraisal process

- The reliability of supervisors in judging standards

- Whether the rating scale produces improved performance and communication

An example of a rating scale and definitions appears in Figure 3.2.

Performance narratives

Performance narratives offer supervisors an opportunity to document their ongoing feedback and evaluation of staff performance. Your goal should be to establish consistency in rating performance across the organization. There is a lot of disagreement regarding what constitutes a good performance evaluation. However, the general thinking is that if you stick to criteria established in your job descriptions, you will make it easier on employees and satisfy surveyors.

FIGURE 3.1

Essential Functions

1. Assesses and diagnoses patient and family needs to provide quality care to assigned patients.

Performs admission assessment within eight hours of admission or in accordance with specific unit standards.

❑ Consistently does not meet standards	❑ Developmental/ needs improvement	❑ Consistently meets/ sometimes exceeds standards	❑ Consistently exceeds standards

Identifies and documents nursing diagnosis on patients' plan of care within eight hours of admission.

❑ Consistently does not meet standards	❑ Developmental/ needs improvement	❑ Consistently meets/ sometimes exceeds standards	❑ Consistently exceeds standards

Identifies and documents patient/family/significant other of admission.

❑ Consistently does not meet standards	❑ Developmental needs improvement	❑ Consistently meets/ sometimes exceeds standards	❑ Consistently exceeds standards

Overall rating

❑ **Consistently does not meet standards**	❑ **Developmental/ needs improvement**	❑ **Consistently meets/sometimes exceeds standards**	❑ **Consistently exceeds standards**

Performance narrative

2. Develops, discusses, and communicates a realistic problem list (plan of care) for each patient, in collaboration with each patient/family/significant other in order to address all identified needs.

Plan of care will include nursing diagnosis statement for each identified problem.

❑ Consistently does not meet standards	❑ Developmental/ needs improvement	❑ Consistently meets/ sometimes exceeds standards	❑ Consistently exceeds standards

Develops patient/family/significant other teaching and discharge plan as per unit standard.

❑ Consistently does not meet standards	❑ Developmental/ needs improvement	❑ Consistently meets/ sometimes exceeds standards	❑ Consistently exceeds standards

Overall rating

❑ **Consistently does not meet standards**	❑ **Developmental/ needs improvement**	❑ **Consistently meets/sometimes exceeds standards**	❑ **Consistently exceeds standards**

Performance narrative

 Competency Management in Long-Term Care

FIGURE 3.2

Rating Scale and Definitions

Consistently exceeds standards	Performance consistently surpasses all established standards. Activities often contribute to improved innovative work practices. This category is to be used for truly outstanding performance.
Consistently meets/ sometimes exceeds standards	Performance meets all established standards and sometimes exceeds them. Activities contribute to increased unit/departmental results. Employees consistently complete the work that is required and at times go beyond expectations.
Developmental/needs improvement	Performance meets most but not all established standards. Activities sometimes contribute to unit/department results. This category is to be used for employees who must demonstrate improvement or more consistent performance and/or for employees still learning their job.
Consistently does not meet standards	Performance is consistently below requirements/expectations. Immediate improvement is necessary.

To this end, a narrative box can be placed at the end of each essential function in your job description (refer to Figure 3.1).

This differs from most traditional performance evaluations, which have space only at the end of the form to document a narrative. This format would allow a supervisor to apply more specific feedback and recommendations.

The key to successfully incorporating your competency assessment process into the ongoing maintenance of job descriptions and the completion of performance evaluations is to develop manageable tools. At the very least, these tools need to identify measurable performance criteria and promote consistent, agreed-upon methods for evaluating the staff (based in part on the populations with which they work) and getting it all done in a timely manner.

REFERENCES

1. Joint Commission Resources. *Comprehensive Accreditation Manual for Hospitals: The Official Handbook.* Oakbrook Terrace, IL: Joint Commission Resources, 2008.

Train the Staff to Perform Competency Validation

Train the Staff to Perform Competency Validation

LEARNING OBJECTIVES

After reading this chapter, the participant should be able to:

✓ Develop a training program to train staff members to perform competency assessments

✓ Maintain consistency in a competency validation system

✓ Identify steps for effective program documentation

✓ Recognize the essential qualities needed by competency assessors

Who performs competency validation within your organization? How are they trained to perform this important responsibility? Ideally, those who assess the competency of others are selected based on their clinical skills and ability to help colleagues enhance job performance. This means they also possess tact and good teaching skills and receive appropriate training prior to evaluating colleagues' job performance. The opposite of this ideal situation is to have all staff members assess the competency of others with little or no training, regardless of their teaching skills.

The truth is that most organizations fall somewhere between these two extremes. The purpose of this chapter is to help you design a practical training program for those staff members responsible for assessing the competency of others.

Developing a Competency Assessment Training Program

Who should be trained to perform competency assessment? First, understand that not all staff members should be trained to assess their colleagues' competency. Competency assessment is an acquired skill that not all healthcare professionals possess.

A competency assessor should possess the following qualifications:

- Excellent performance of the competencies being evaluated

- Tact and the desire to help colleagues improve their job performance

- The desire to acquire/enhance adult education skills

- Demonstration of excellent interpersonal communication skills

Now that you know who should be trained, what should you include in the training program? The following components should be part of your competency assessment training and education program.

Purpose

Learners need to understand the purpose and importance of a competency assessment program. You need to be able to demonstrate how job performance is enhanced and resident care improved by adhering to competency criteria. Use quality improvement and risk management data to prove your point. Learners must also understand that the public health department, The Joint Commission, Centers for Medicare & Medicaid Services, and other accrediting agencies expect staff members to demonstrate their competence, that such competence is evaluated on an ongoing basis, and that each staff member's competence is documented.

Principles of adult learning

Any educational program that involves training adults to teach/coach other adults must include an overview of the principles of adult learning (Avillion, Brunt, and Ferrell 2007). For example:

- **Adults must have a valid reason for learning.** Adults want proof that there is a need for learning (i.e., they want to know why it is important for them to participate in an educational activity). For example, suppose the ability to perform a sterile dressing change is a competency for all RNs. Some of them complain that they perform this task frequently and they don't need someone observing them to validate their competency. If you are able to cite quality improvement data indicating a negative trend (e.g., infections) due to questionable techniques, you can show them why there is a need for continual competency assessment. National data can also be cited to illustrate the need for keeping on top of a particular skill.

- **Adults are self-directed learners.** Adults direct their own learning. They want to feel that they have some control over what they learn and the manner in which they learn it. Adults also need to feel that their opinions matter and their learning needs are respected.

- **Adults bring a variety of life experiences to any learning situation.** Such life experiences can facilitate any learning activity. Even experiences not directly related to healthcare can enhance education.

- **Adults concentrate on acquiring knowledge and skills that help them improve their professional and/or personal lives.** Adults measure the importance of education by focusing on how new knowledge and skills will help them improve their professional performance or enhance their private lives.

- **Adults respond to extrinsic and intrinsic motivators.** Adults must know how learning activities meet their extrinsic and intrinsic needs. Extrinsic motivators include incentives such as job promotions and salary raises. Examples of intrinsic motivators include enhanced self-esteem and an increase in job satisfaction.

Learning styles

When you assess competency, you are often in a teaching position. Even though a staff member demonstrates competency, you may have suggestions to help improve some aspect of his or her skill. Include an overview of the following types of learners when you design your competency assessment training program (Avillion 2004):

- **Auditory learners** assimilate knowledge by hearing. They prefer lectures, discussions, and audiotapes. They respond most favorably to verbal instructions.

- **Visual learners** are the most common type of adult learners. They sit in the front of a classroom, take detailed notes, and respond to verbal discussions that contain a lot of imagery.

- **Kinesthetic learners** learn best by doing. They need direct hands-on involvement and physical activity as part of the learning experience.

Maintaining objectivity

It is important that those who assess competency maintain their objectivity. The training program should contain information about performing objective evaluations and not letting personal feelings—positive or negative—influence the outcome of the assessment.

Offering constructive criticism

This is one of the most challenging responsibilities of anyone who evaluates the job performance of others. The purpose of constructive criticism is to provide feedback on strengths and weaknesses. Constructive criticism should motivate, reinforce learning, and identify the nature and extent of problems. One of the most important parts of constructive criticism is the development of a specific plan to help staff members improve their performance. Use the following four steps when giving feedback:

1. **Identify the unacceptable actions.** What is the staff member doing or failing to do that is not acceptable? Remember to focus on the employee's behavior, not on his or her personality. Give specific examples, such as "You did not follow sterile techniques when you touched the soiled wound dressing with your sterile-gloved hand," not "It seems as though you do not care whether you endanger the resident by ignoring proper sterile techniques."

2. **Explain the outcome.** Why is the behavior unacceptable? How does it negatively affect productivity, resident outcomes, and so on? Be specific. Use descriptive terms instead of evaluative terms.

3. **Establish the expectation.** What must the employee do to correct unacceptable behavior? Again, be specific and use objective, descriptive terms. You are describing actions

to improve behavior, not providing evalua-tive comments about a person's personality.

4. **Identify the consequences.** What will hap-pen if the employee corrects his or her behavior? What will happen if he or she does not?

How to assess competency consistently

One of the biggest challenges of any competency assessment program is the need for consistency among those conducting the assessments. How do you make sure that one person is not too stringent and another too lenient? Are friends assessing friends' competency? Does this make a difference in the outcome? Are people who dislike each other assessing each other's competency? Your training program must provide staff members with the tools and support needed to conduct competency assessments properly. This includes maintaining up-to-date policies and procedures, appropriate documentation checklists, and adequate education and training (a detailed description of these com-ponents appears later in this chapter).

Consistency in documentation is as important as consistency in approach. Everyone should use the same tool template. A procedure that describes how to document competency is needed.

Identifying Your Competency Assessors

Can you identify competency assessors by title? Let's look at the following common job titles that may carry with them the responsibility for compe-tency assessment:

- **Nurse managers, supervisors, and precep-tors.** The ability to perform competency assessment is an integral role of nursing leadership in long-term care. A preceptor is an excellent method to promote a successful orientation of new employees. The essential qualities needed by competency assessors are also key leadership attributes. These qualities include:

  – Possessing excellent clinical skills or, in non-clinical roles, excellence in job-specific skills

  – Demonstrating respect for colleagues

  – Acting as an excellent role model

  – Demonstrating outstanding interpersonal communication skills

To increase the efficiency of training delivery and orientation, consider inviting staff members who need to be trained as competency assessors to a class that offers training in competency assess-ment. Directors of nursing (DON) are generally not the best people to assess clinical competency. In today's healthcare environment, DONs spend most of their time performing administrative duties such as staffing, budgeting, developing lead-ership, and handling performance issues. However, their expertise in these areas makes them able to validate such competencies in their nursing lead-ership team. DONs rely on their staff members to possess clinical expertise, just as staff members rely on the DON for administrative expertise. Remember that to assess clinical competency properly, the evaluator must be able to demon-strate excellence in clinical skills. Most DONs in long-term care will be able to demonstrate these clinical skills but are not the ones delivering the care on a daily basis. DONs assess the supervisory and leadership skill competency of their nurse management team.

- **Directors of staff development (DSDs)** are the education experts in a long-term care facility.

  They must demonstrate competency in the adult education and clinical skills arenas. Such competencies as program planning, teaching, and evaluating the effectiveness of education are essential to those who specialize in staff development.

  Staff development specialists work with management and the staff to design the organization's entire competency assessment program in addition to the program's training component. They provide the educational expertise that makes for a sound foundation for any competency program. But like anyone who is responsible for assessing competency, staff development specialists must be competent in the skills they evaluate.

- **Staff nurses.** Nurses who demonstrate the necessary skills may also be part of a competency assessment program. However, it is important that they receive the necessary training. Depending on the arrangement of your clinical ladder or other similar programs, you may choose to have competency assessment as part of the requirements for promotion.

- **Certified nursing assistants (CNA).** Can you think of exceptionally competent CNAs in your organization? Training such CNAs to assess the competency of their peers is a definite possibility. As you develop a promotional

ladder for CNAs, consider training those who are exceptional to participate in competency assessment.

- **Nonclinical staff.** Most healthcare organizations have competency assessment programs in place for clinical and nonclinical areas. As your competency program develops and expands, don't forget to be on the lookout for nonclinical staff members who have what it takes to assess the competency of others in areas such as fire safety.

You already know that you need to document competency achievement. Don't forget to document that your trainees have achieved competency in their ability to evaluate the performance of others. Figure 4.1 shows an example of a form you can use for such documentation.

Keeping Your Validation System Consistent

Nothing is as demoralizing as inconsistency in evaluation, and few things are as challenging as ensuring consistency of approach among many people. The following are some tips for maintaining inter-rater reliability among your competency assessors:

- Make sure that the assessor has the ability to assess the competency of fellow employees. Successful completion of the training program on competency assessment must be documented. Failure to successfully complete the program demands that the trainee perform remedial work. He or she must not assess the competency of others until training is successfully completed.

FIGURE 4.1

Successful Completion of Competency Assessment Training Form

Date: _____

Objectives: _____

_____

_____

Competency demonstration:
1. Explains purpose and importance of a competency assessment program
2. Incorporates the principles of adult learning as part of assessing competency
3. Recognizes various learning styles and meets the needs of learners representing these styles
4. Maintains objectivity when assessing competency
5. Offers feedback in a constructive manner
6. Is consistent in competency assessment approach
7. Documents results of competency assessment accurately and consistently

Trainer comments:

_____

_____

_____

Learner comments:

_____

_____

_____

Competency assessment training was successfully completed:

_____   _____
 Trainer's signature and date   Learner's signature and date

Competency assessment training was not successfully completed:

_____
 Trainer's signature and date

The following steps will be taken by the learner to successfully complete training:

    Action: To be completed by the following date:

_____

_____

_____

_____
 Learner's signature and date

- Avoid compromising objectivity whenever possible. If competency is assessed individually in an on-the-job environment, avoid pairing staff members who have known interpersonal conflicts. Likewise, avoid pairing staff members who are close friends. Either situation runs the risk of accusations of prejudice or favoritism. Doing so may enhance objectivity.

- Ensure that the steps that must be performed, along with descriptions regarding how they are to be performed, are clearly documented on the competency assessment form. Never assume that everyone knows how to do a certain competency. Failure to achieve competency can have dramatic consequences, including termination of employment. The only way to ensure consistency fairly is to provide a written guide delineating what constitutes successful competency demonstration.

- Develop a written checklist so that competency is evaluated on a step-by-step basis. The competency assessor must sign and date the checklist. The learner must also sign and date the checklist. Any remedial action plans must be documented along with targeted dates for achievement.

- Require the person assessing competency to document his or her evaluation findings. This task cannot be delegated to someone else. For example, suppose a busy manager asks one of her senior staff nurses to document a competency assessment for her. This is completely unacceptable. Competency assessment is just like any other type of nursing documentation: If you do it, you document it.

- Have a plan in place to deal with persons who object to their competency rating. Include this plan in your policies and procedures. If a staff member is unfairly evaluated, he or she needs to know that there is a professional way to seek a reassessment. The steps that must be taken, including any necessary objective evidence, should be described in these policies and procedures.

- Ensure that policies and procedures describe the circumstances under which a grievance or other protest mechanism will be heard.

Incorporating Population-Specific Competencies

The various physiological and psychological needs of each resident are part of any well-designed person-centered competency program. The ability to implement individualized interventions is critical to the quality and suitability of resident care.

What are some efficient, cost-effective ways to achieve and demonstrate population-specific competencies? Let's start with education and training.

Simply attending an educational program does not guarantee transfer of learning to the work setting. However, because healthcare science and research seems to bring new and exciting discoveries to the healthcare arena every day, part of the requirement of competency maintenance may involve participating in a specified number of age-specific educational hours. These hours do not need to be offered exclusively in a classroom setting. Options such as self-learning packets, videos, and computer-based learning are cost-effective, efficient ways to deliver education and training. Successful achievement of educational posttests measures learning or the acquisition of knowledge.

But as we discussed earlier in this chapter, knowledge acquisition does not equate to the ability to successfully transfer knowledge. How can we assess population-specific competencies? Ongoing competency may be evaluated in several ways, including direct observation, medical record review, and outcomes. Let's review the competency of Melanie, a nurse who works with frail, elderly residents with dementia. We can use the following methodologies to be sure that she is competent in providing care to people with dementia:

- **Medical record review:** Are appropriate nursing interventions documented? Is there documented evidence that safety measures are in place considering the resident's diagnosis? Identify specific interventions for the assessor to find within the medical record, including nursing care plans, nurses' notes, and so on. You need to be specific to facilitate consistency of evaluation.

- **Direct observations:** Does Melanie provide care in a manner that incorporates population-specific concerns for the person with dementia? In addition to observing Melanie as she actually provides care, you can assess outcomes and the environment. For example, when assessing safety issues, determine whether the walker is within reach, whether nonskid slippers are readily available, and so on. Again, be specific about what assessors need to evaluate. Select some specific dementia care communication and approach guidelines and determine whether these interventions are part of the resident's care plan.

- **Equipment use:** Is equipment use adapted to the needs of the person with dementia? For example, if a resident with dementia requires a mechanical lift for transferring, are measures taken to avoid potential dangers such as skin tears, bruises, and agitation?

These are only a few of the ways to assess population-specific competency. Remember that all reviewers must carry out such assessments in a consistent manner. This means that written guidelines must be established.

Documentation and Recordkeeping

It is essential that your competency assessment program include appropriate documentation and maintenance of such documentation. Various sample checklists and templates are presented throughout this chapter. As a summary of important issues, let's review the following essential documentation components:

- **Assessment documentation must be dated.** Although you may think that this component is self-evident, it is astonishing how many times it is missed. The top of any form generally contains a space for the date, but all signatures should be dated as well. This decreases the chance of any discrepancies concerning assessment dates.

- **Identify the specific competency being assessed.** This includes specifying the population being assessed in the population-specific competencies.

- **Identify both the behavioral objectives and performance objectives that must be** achieved to demonstrate competency. These objectives should be written in measurable terms and contain action verbs such as performs, identifies, and demonstrates. Nonmeasurable terms, such as "understand" and "be aware of," are to be avoided.

- **Document specific steps in competency achievement.** Consistency cannot be ensured unless the specific, step-by-step actions that must be performed to achieve competency are in writing. All assessors must have the same expectations of the people they are evaluating.

- **Document the methods used to assess competency.** Possible methods include observation of direct resident care, medical record review, and evaluation of the resident's environment. Again, don't forget to identify what the assessor must look for in the selected methods.

- **Document remedial action.** If competency is not achieved, document the remedial actions that will be taken to help the learner achieve competency. The actions should be specific and should include target achievement dates.

Conclusion

Competency assessment is an integral part of your resident care. Those who assess the competency of others must receive appropriate education and training so that they are effective, efficient, and consistent in their approach.

Careful objective documentation of such education and training is as important as documentation of competency assessment itself. In fact, achievement as a competency assessor is a competency too. Carefully select those individuals who assess competency. Not every staff member is suited to assess and facilitate learning in others. Clinical excellence does not equate to the ability to facilitate the job performance of colleagues.

The templates and forms presented in this chapter are intended to be starting points for the customization of your own tools. Adapt them to meet the needs of your staff members.

Finally, remember that competency assessment is a learning tool as well as a means of validation. Use these opportunities to facilitate the continuing education and professional development of staff members, with the ultimate goal being improved resident outcomes.

REFERENCES

1. Agnes, Michael (Ed). *Webster's New World College Dictionary*. Cleveland: Wiley Publishing, 2006.

2. Avillion, Adrianne E. *A Practical Guide to Staff Development: Tools and Techniques for Effective Education*. Marblehead, MA: HCPro, Inc., 2004.

3. Avillion, Adrianne E., Brunt, Barbara A., and Ferrell, Mary Jane. *Nursing Professional Development Review and Resource Manual*. Silver Spring, MD: Institute for Credentialing Innovation, 2007.

Keep Up with
New Competencies

Keep Up with New Competencies

After reading this chapter, the participant should be able to:

✓ List potential categories for new competencies

✓ Identify best practices for implementing new competencies

✓ Discuss dimensions of competencies

Hundreds of new concerns arise in healthcare daily. How do you determine which ones become competencies?

Let's start by describing what a competency is not. Competencies are not required for every new piece of equipment, new or revised policy and procedure, interpersonal communication problem, or skill that accompanies a specific job description. However, a competency is a skill that significantly affects or has the potential to significantly affect the resident. Such issues may fall under the categories of psychomotor skills or interpersonal skills.

Doesn't everything in healthcare have the potential to significantly affect a resident? Technically, yes. But if you define the word "significant" that broadly, you will have so many competencies that you'll drown in paperwork, and it will become impossible to assess that many items efficiently.

Potential Categories for New Competencies

Let's look at some general categories that have the potential for competency development.

New equipment

Not every piece of new equipment triggers the need for a competency. In most cases, a simple inservice suffices. For example, suppose your organization orders new beds. The beds have some additional features that the old beds lacked, and an inservice is conducted to orient staff members to work safely with these new beds. Now suppose that new equipment, including Circoelectric beds, Bradford frames, and Stryker frames, arrives for your organization's newly opened rehabilitation unit. These devices require special skills to ensure safety and will be used often, although not daily. These types of new equipment are more suitable for ongoing competency development. They significantly affect the patient, require a high level of skill and safety awareness, and are used frequently.

When new equipment arrives, ask yourself the following questions:

- Does the equipment require high levels of skill to operate?

- Who will operate the new equipment? Must the staff have special qualifications (e.g., RN designation) to use this equipment?

- What potential resident safety risks are associated with the new equipment?

- How often will the new equipment be in use?

If you find that equipment requires qualified staff members to have high levels of skill, is associated with significant resident safety issues, and is used often enough that the staff is able to maintain competency, the equipment may require the development of a competency.

Interpersonal Communication

Interpersonal communication is the foundation of healthcare interventions. From the first contact at a reception desk or admission's office through and including communication with physicians, nurses, social workers, certified nursing assistants, recreation therapists, housekeeping, and the dietary staff, interpersonal interaction influences the residents' daily life. For the people who have cognitive loss, our interpersonal communication skills need to be altered to meet their needs.

How would you rate interpersonal communication skills among your colleagues? Does risk management/quality improvement data indicate any negative trends in this arena? Do staff members encounter hostility from residents or families? How do you assess this type of competency? It is not a step-by-step psychomotor skill. However, there are options.

Direct observation is one such option; however, keep in mind that written guidelines are necessary for the person assessing competency. Additional observations may be set up in a competency skills lab, where staff members must respond to various types of behavior in role-play situations. These are not conducted in the actual work setting, but they may be a useful addendum to direct observation.

Be creative when assessing nontechnical skills such as these. Another validation option is to conduct mock drills involving staff members playing the role of agitated/violent residents or family members. Mock drills have the advantage of surprise and may be more valuable than a controlled role-play situation.

New patient populations

The appearance of new diseases and syndromes requires the implementation of new diagnostic and treatment interventions. The AIDS epidemic changed almost every aspect of healthcare and triggered the need for universal precautions and more secure protective equipment. The development of new drugs to combat this syndrome requires that healthcare professionals add to the ever-growing body of knowledge concerning medications, their actions, and potential side effects. The number of residents with obesity is growing every year. Caring for a bariatric population requires the staff to have specific knowledge related to the needs of this population.

New patient populations require new knowledge and the application of that knowledge in the healthcare setting. As you evaluate the need for new skills to apply this knowledge, you are also evaluating the need for additional competency development. However, stick to the recommendations made earlier in this chapter. Consider the level of knowledge and skill needed, how often the knowledge will be applied, and the effect of these newly acquired skills on patient outcomes.

New treatment measures

Thanks to intense research and scientific inquiry, we are able to treat and even cure illnesses and catastrophic injuries that were untreatable just a few short years ago. With these healthcare advances come new bodies of knowledge and the need to use that knowledge safely and efficiently. As new treatment measures become necessary to your organization's ability to provide services, so does the need for additional competency development. Remember that you don't need to keep the same

competencies forever. Perhaps new treatments and equipment and the demise or reduction of certain illnesses trigger the need for you to delete certain competencies from your program. As you evaluate the need for new competencies, don't forget to evaluate the need to streamline those already in existence.

New medications

The FDA approves significant numbers of new medications annually. Most of them do not require competency development; however, some drugs require special knowledge, and administration techniques for these drugs necessitate competency development. Use your guidelines of skill level, resident impact, and frequency of use to determine the need for new competencies.

Research endeavors

If your facility is a research site, your staff members may be exposed to new (and sometimes dangerous) ways of treating illnesses and injuries more often than the average healthcare worker. Examine your research policies and procedures. Which staff members frequently initiate experimental treatments, including medication administration? How do you measure their competency to initiate these treatments? As you evaluate your competency assessment program, don't forget to pay close attention to the research conducted at your organization: The resultant treatment initiatives could mandate the development of new competencies.

Guidelines for New Competency Development

Develop a policy that guides your competency assessment program (Avillion 2004). Part of that

---

policy describes your guidelines for new competency development and for the deletion of competencies that are no longer necessary.

Answer the following questions to identify what to incorporate into your facility's policy:

- What new procedure diagnostic tests or treatments have been developed that require staff members to add to their knowledge and expertise?

- What current competencies no longer meet the criteria for ongoing competency assessment? Are the treatments outdated, are they no longer initiated, or have they become part of a daily routine with reduced effect on resident outcome and little or no exceptional level of skill?

- What level of skill do new initiatives require?

- Who is authorized to perform/evaluate the effectiveness of new initiatives?

- What safety risks to residents, visitors, and staff members are associated with these new initiatives?

- How often will these new initiatives be implemented?

Think about your answer to the last question carefully. Staff members cannot achieve or retain competency unless they have fairly regular opportunities to use new knowledge and skills.

The checklist in Figure 5.1 may help you document your assessment of the need for new competency development.

FIGURE 5.1

New Competency Assessment Checklist

Date: _____

Item being evaluated:

- ❏ New equipment
- ❏ New treatment
- ❏ New medication

- ❏ New resident population
- ❏ Interpersonal communication issue
- ❏ Research initiatives

Identify the item specifically (e.g., type and purpose of equipment and description of new treatment).

_____

_____

1. What new knowledge/skills are required to safely initiate this new item?

_____

_____

2. Who is authorized to perform these new skills (e.g., RNs or LPNs?)

_____

_____

3. What, if any, quality improvement/risk management data indicate a need for this competency?

_____

_____

4. What risks to patients, visitors, and staff members are associated with the new initiative?

_____

_____

5. How often will staff members have an opportunity to apply the new knowledge and skills necessary for safe, accurate implementation of this new initiative?

_____

_____

There is a need for new competency development. The new competency is:

_____

_____

_____

Signature, title, and date

There is no need for new competency development. The rationale for this is:

_____

_____

_____

Signature, title, and date

Best Practices for the Implementation of New Competencies

Unfortunately, new competencies do not evolve neatly on an annual basis, allowing ample time for appropriate education and training to occur. They pop up at any time, with varying degrees of urgency. The following are some suggestions for implementing new competencies (Cooper 2002).

Competency skills fairs

Some organizations have implemented daylong or half-day competency assessments. These are called by various names, such as skills fairs, competency days, and competency skills labs. The premise is generally the same: A variety of competencies are assessed during a specified period and at an identified general location (usually a classroom setting). These events can be held annually, semiannually, or quarterly.

Advantages of this approach include:

- **Efficiency.** Competency days allow you to address the maximum number of people with a minimum number of observers.

- **Regular scheduling.** Staff members know when these events will occur and, in conjunction with their managers, can plan their attendance. Likewise, those responsible for organizing the competency days have planning time and the chance to add/delete competencies.

- **Decreased time away from the actual work site.** By planning regular assessment days, staffing needs can be planned in advance.

Disadvantages of this approach include:

- Competencies are added or deleted only at specific times throughout the year. This may compromise the timeliness of critical competency assessments.

- Competencies that require demonstration of actual care interactions/procedures are not suitable for this approach.

- There may be an insufficient number of competency assessors on hand.

- Determining the length of time the fair is open. Twenty-four-hour availability requires a lot of competency assessors. If 24-hour availability is not possible, determining the hours of operation can draw complaints from staff members who must attend on their time off. In addition, because competency assessment is a mandate, the organization must pay for staff members to attend, which can place a considerable burden on the budget.

Drills and simulations

An evaluation form must be completed after each drill. This form serves as a record of behavior, a competency assessment, and a format to document strengths and areas for improvement.

Examples of drills and simulations include mock codes, internal and external disasters, and hazardous-spill cleanup.

Drills and simulations:

- Require little or no additional staffing

- Can serve as a complement to the annual review of the environment of care plans required by the Occupational Safety & Health Administration

- Evaluate behavior in true-life situations

Disadvantages of drills and simulations are that they:

- May disrupt other programs or upset the residents' activities

- Require exceptionally detail-oriented evaluators

- Need specific identification of required behaviors on evaluation forms

Performance improvement monitors

This approach relies on data from performance improvement (PI) documentation. PI indicators are useful when evaluating interpersonal competencies and abilities to perform clinical skills.

Advantages of using PI monitors include the following:

- PI monitors are regular, reliable sources of data

- No additional time burden is required to collect the data

- Managers can simultaneously validate competency and complete a mandated activity without additional work, making the process more efficient

Disadvantages of using PI monitors include the following:

- They require the assumption that the PI data are accurate and objective

- They do not guarantee that competency was consistently evaluated if multiple people had input into the performance evaluation

Return demonstration/observation

Return demonstration can take place during the previously mentioned skills fair or on the job, which involves direct observation of skill performance.

Demonstration/observation allows:

- The assessor to actually see behavior and the employee's application of knowledge

- For demonstration of new knowledge and skills in the actual work environment in real-life settings

Disadvantages of return demonstration/observation include the following:

- It may influence the behavior of the staff member being assessed because he or she is aware that an evaluation is taking place

- It cannot guarantee that the employee's behavior is the same during the return demonstration/observation as when not being observed

Self-assessment

Self-assessment generally requires that employees complete a written exercise designed to identify their beliefs and knowledge about their job performance. An employee's assessment is compared to the manager's and other assessors' assessments.

Any disparity must be addressed so that job performance improves.

Advantages of self-assessment include the following:

- Helps employees recognize their beliefs and values and how these issues may affect their job performance

- Identifies incongruence between employees' beliefs and values and the organization's mission, vision, and values

Disadvantages of self-assessment include the following:

- Does not provide an opportunity for evaluation of actual behaviors

- Only provides results that are influenced by employees' and assessors' personal values and beliefs

- Does not address incongruence results in employees continuing to behave in ways that are inconsistent with the organization's mission, vision, and values

Dimensions of Competencies

Each approach is distinct and focuses on specific aspects of employee skills. According to *Competency Assessment: A Practical Guide to the JCAHO Standards,* 2nd Edition (Summers et al 2004), competencies are designed to evaluate particular features of skills, called dimensions. Each dimension includes explicit skills and knowledge, including:

- Critical-thinking dimension—the ability to use information or knowledge, including:

  - Problem solving

  - Planning

  - Clinical reasoning

  - Adapting to/facilitating change

  - Time management

  - Fiscal responsibility

- Interpersonal dimension—the ability to work effectively with others, including:

  - Communication

  - Conflict management

  - Customer service

  - Work effectively with members of various cultures and racial and ethnic backgrounds

- Technical dimension—the possession of knowledge and the ability to use that knowledge to perform fine and gross motor functions, including:

  - Cognitive abilities

  - Acquired knowledge

  - Psychomotor ability

  - Technical competence

As you evaluate the need for new competencies, review these dimensions to determine need and approach. Remember that a competency assessment program focuses on verifying and validating skills and knowledge application in the workplace. The purpose of a competency program is to:

- Improve job performance

- Enhance patient outcomes

- Promote economic efficiency

- Increase organizational effectiveness

Demonstrated achievement of these goals shows that your competency assessment program is one that not only validates knowledge and skills, but also results in improved patient outcomes.

REFERENCES

1. Avillion, Adrianne E., *A Practical Guide to Staff Development: Tools and Techniques for Effective Education.* Marblehead, MA: HCPro, Inc., 2004.

2. Cooper, D. "The 'C' Word: Competency." *Staff Development Nursing Secrets.* Philadelphia: Hanley & Belfus, 2002.

3. Summers, B., Tracy, J., and Woods, W. *Competency Assessment: A Practical Guide to the JCAHO Standards,* 2nd Edition. Marblehead, MA: HCPro, Inc., 2004.

Using Your Skills
Checklists

Using Your Skills Checklists

Skills checklists must clearly identify expectations and should be completed by staff members who know how to use them. Criteria for safe, effective performance must be clearly defined, and everyone participating in the evaluation process must have a common understanding of the criteria and the basis for assigning ratings. Research has shown that making direct observations using precise measurement criteria in checklists, with immediate feedback on performance, is more effective than the traditional evaluation of clinical skills using subjective rating forms. The format for skills checklists may vary, but most contain similar information. Regardless of how they are used, skills checklists should:

- Be learner-oriented

- Focus on behaviors

- Be measurable

- Use criteria validated by experts

- Be specific enough to avoid ambiguity

A template used to create the skills checklists included in this manual appears in Figure 6.1, and an electronic version of this template appears on your accompanying CD-ROM; you can open it as a Microsoft Word document. The individual's name and date are important to identify whose skills are being validated and when the evaluation is being conducted.

The steps identified in the checklist should define the critical behaviors needed for effective performance of the skill and do not include every step of the procedure. You can use the "Completed" column to indicate that each step was performed correctly, but note that some checklists use a "Met/Not met" format instead. It is helpful if checklists include an area for comments. Also note that most checklists are used to evaluate one occurrence.

In the checklist format just described, the self-assessment can give the evaluator an idea of the individual's perceived skill level, although that can never take the place of validating competency. Individuals may have different perceptions of their abilities that may or may not be consistent with the evaluator's perceptions. For example, one person could indicate that she needs practice, even though she is familiar and competent with that skill, but is not familiar with the institution's policy and procedure. Another staff member could indicate that he needs practice because he has performed the skill only once during his career. All required skills must be validated, regardless of an individual's assessment of his or her ability.

The evaluation/validation method areas indicate how the validation was performed. The method used most often is demonstration or observation of the individual performing the skill, but verbal questioning can also be effective in identifying the thought processes or critical thinking involved with skills. Practical exercises and interactive class activities can also be useful as validation methods.

The appropriate level (beginner, intermediate, or expert) can be indicated, as well as the type of validation. It is important to identify whether the assessment is part of an individual's orientation or whether it is an ongoing annual validation. It is also important that you have the employee and the observer sign the checklist.

The Joint Commission mandates that all employees have their competence assessed upon hire and throughout their employment. One way to meet this standard is to have orientation checklists in addition to skills checklists (Joint Commission Resources 2008).

Differences between Orientation Checklists and Skills Checklists

Orientation checklists specify the knowledge, attitudes, and skills needed to perform safely. The information for an orientation checklist would come from the position description for that job classification and would outline the essential competencies for safe practice in that role. Skills checklists, on the other hand, include the specific tasks related to a policy or procedure. Skills checklists are often used to document ongoing competency, as compared to orientation checklists, which document initial competency.

Developing orientation checklists

Key elements in developing an orientation checklist are the job description and performance evaluation criteria. The components of the orientation program provide the framework. Essential information in the checklist would include the individual's name and the names of all evaluators. The hire date and unit are helpful to identify when the individual started in his or her role. Orientation checklists provide documentation of the initial assessment of competence as well as the individual's self-assessment. If evaluation during the orientation is a shared responsibility (e.g., with directors of staff development and nurse managers or preceptors), different columns can be used to identify what was done during a classroom orientation and what was done on the units. A "Not Evaluated" or "Not Applicable" column can be helpful for those skills that an employee did not have an opportunity to develop during the orientation process.

Sample checklists for RN orientation (Figure 6.2) and CNA orientation (Figure 6.3) are included as examples.

Orientation checklists should be developed with input from the management staff. This will ensure that they include the essential skills expected from the position. Generally, staff development, nurse managers, supervisors, or preceptors complete orientation checklists. Preceptors help new employees adjust to the unit, introduce them to the residents, and work with new employees to help plan the learning experiences and share knowledge of expected behaviors. They can help reduce stress and enhance learning for new employees by using adult-learning principles, documenting skill acquisition, and helping the new person acclimate to the facility's culture. The checklist helps to make employees accountable for their learning by clearly identifying expectations to be completed during the orientation period. After the orientation checklist is completed, it usually becomes part of the employee's permanent file, which protects the employer and the employee.

Skills Checklists for Annual Competency Assessment

This section provides suggestions on how to determine which skills to evaluate, develop the skills checklists, identify who can complete the checklists, and keep track of who has been evaluated. It also reviews what happens if someone does not meet identified competencies, and it includes a brief discussion of other methods of validating competence.

Determining which skills to evaluate

Your facility needs to set up a system to determine which competencies to evaluate each year. Chapter 2 provided a suggested formula to use when determining which skills to evaluate. There is no right or wrong way to select the skills to be evaluated, as long as the facility can justify why the particular skills were chosen. Skills should be selected based on the individual needs of the unit or facility.

Developing the skills checklists

Once the skills to be assessed are selected, skills checklists can be developed or modified from the samples attached to ensure consistency in evaluation. Review your facility's policies and procedures using current literature for support. The essential steps of the policies and procedures are incorporated into the skills checklists, many of which you can easily adapt for your needs by changing the criteria to be consistent with steps in your policies and procedures or standards.

Identifying who can complete the checklists

It is important to identify who (e.g., what job classification) can validate skills for each job classification. It may be better to have an RN or licensed practical nurse check off a CNA on vital signs rather than have another CNA complete the skills check-list. Individuals who are responsible for validating someone's skill should be qualified based on education, experience, or expertise with that skill, or they should have already demonstrated proficiency with that skill. Individuals with documented competence in the skill they are validating should assess ongoing competence. That competence may be determined by his or her role (e.g., advanced practice nurse, staff development nurse, nurse manager, or supervisor), frequency of performing the skill, or already having demonstrated competence in that skill.

When introducing new technology or procedures into the clinical area, individuals with documented experience in that procedure (e.g., physicians, nurses from that specialty, or vendor representatives) should perform the initial training. A core group of staff members or a single individual can be trained and confirm the competency of other staff members after they personally demonstrate competence in that skill.

Keeping track of who has been evaluated

Each evaluator should refer to the skills checklist when observing a staff member perform that skill. Skills checklists for the competencies being evaluated can be kept in a competency notebook as a reference for the staff. These checklists can be used to assess initial and ongoing competence. The use of a checklist ensures consistency in evaluating the steps to perform the skill. Rather than completing an individual skills checklist for every person evaluated, a tracking sheet can typically be used to document completion of that skill.

The tracking sheet provides a way to document that staff members in each classification have completed required competencies. Names of the unit staff members are written on the tracking sheet, and when someone is checked off on a particular competency, the individual observing that person writes in the date and his or her initials in the column for that particular competency in the row with that person's name. Individuals are responsible for ensuring that someone validates their required skills each year. The manager then uses this information when completing performance appraisals.

The Competencies Analyzer

Figure 6.4 provides a sample tracking sheet. We've also provided an electronic version of this Excel spreadsheet on your accompanying CD-ROM. The Competencies Analyzer is an easy way for a manager to track competency assessment.

Determining what happens when a staff member cannot perform competencies

Facilities need to identify the consequences when a staff member cannot demonstrate mastery of a competency. Policies may vary, but a mechanism needs to be in place to safeguard residents and ensure that the staff member is not assigned to a resident who requires that competency. Possible options would be to provide remediation and further clinical experiences or to transfer the staff member to another area where he or she can meet the required competencies. Continued failure to demonstrate required competencies may lead to a plan for improvement or termination.

Other methods to validate competence

It is also important to realize that the skills checklists are only one method to validate competence; other methods may be used. Some skills may not happen frequently enough to check all staff members off on that skill, and skills fairs may be an alternative approach. During skills fairs, employees are tested and validated on skills using simulations, games, word puzzles, or other methods to verify that they are aware of the steps of the procedure. Skills checklists can also be used during fairs for those skills that may not come up frequently enough to check everyone on a unit.

With the increasing sophistication of technology, computer-assisted video evaluation may be used to evaluate competency in a particular area. Videotaped or simulated scenarios can give evaluators the opportunity to observe and rate performances. With this approach, ratings can be compared with the instructor to clarify any discrepancies and determine inter-rater reliability. However, this may not be realistic in organizations where many staff members will be completing skills checklists for their peers.

One problem with skills checklists is that you don't know whether the observed behavior is persistent and representative of the situation being observed, or whether the individual is going through the correct steps knowing that someone is evaluating him or her for that single occurrence. Therefore, indirect observation can also be used. Often, managers or charge nurses conduct rounds and medical record reviews. With indirect observation, there may not be direct observation of the skills, but there is the presumption that the skills are correctly followed when the desired outcomes are achieved. Clinical rounds can measure competencies as well as improve the standard of care and practice in the clinical setting.

Facilities need to have a competency-based program in place to ensure that individuals are prepared to deliver quality resident care. Assessment of competency begins with orientation and continues throughout employment. An evaluation of each nursing staff member's competency should be conducted at defined intervals throughout the individual's association with the facility. Performance appraisals and skills checklists may be used to measure the ongoing competency of nursing employees. Continuing education programs and inservices can also enhance staff members' competency.

Competence assessment for nursing staff members and volunteers who provide direct resident care is based on:

- Populations served, including age ranges and specialties

- Competencies required for role and provision of care

- Competencies assessed during orientation

- Unit-specific competencies that need to be assessed or reassessed annually based on care modalities, age ranges, techniques, procedures, technology, equipment, skills needed, or changes in laws and regulations

- Appropriate assessment methods for the skill being assessed

- Delineation of who is qualified to assess competence

- A description of action taken when improvement activities lead to a determination that a staff member with performance problems is unable or unwilling to improve

Individuals who transfer from another area in the facility know which competencies they must meet at the time of their orientation.

The following is a list of some questions to consider in an evaluation of the competence assessment system (Cooper 2002):

- Is the new-employee competence assessment completed during the initial orientation process?

- Is employee orientation based on assessed competencies and the knowledge and skills required to deliver resident care services?

- Is the new-employee competence assessment completed at the conclusion of the orientation process?

- Do clinical staff members participate in ongoing educational activities to acquire new competencies that support resident care delivery? Are those activities minimally based on quality improvement findings, new technology, therapeutic or pharmacology interventions, and the learning needs of the nursing staff?

- Does the management or leadership staff participate in competence assessment activities (i.e., clinical knowledge, skills, or technology)?

- Does the management or leadership staff participate in ongoing education activities to acquire new competencies for resident care management (i.e., management development)?

- Does the performance evaluation system address staff competence?

- When competency deficiencies are noted, is a plan for correction initiated and implemented?

- Does reassessment of competence occur as necessary?

- Are summaries of competence assessment findings available by individual, resident-care unit, and department?

- Are plans for competence maintenance and improvement documented?

- Is an annual report submitted to the governing body?

- Do policies and procedures exist to define the process of competence assessment?

The overall competence assessment process must be reviewed on an ongoing basis to determine its effectiveness and any opportunities for improvement. This evaluation identifies what works, what doesn't, why it doesn't, and how it can be improved. It can take a very formal approach through survey methodology and interviews or a less formal approach of asking for subjective data and feedback from key people and groups.

REFERENCES

1. Joint Commission Resources. *Comprehensive Accreditation Manual for Hospitals: The Official Handbook.* Oakbrook, IL: Joint Commission Resources, 2008.

2. Cooper, D. "The 'C' Word: Competency." *Staff Development Nursing Secrets.* Philadelphia: Hanley & Belfus, 2002.

FIGURE 6.1

Skills Checklist Template

Name: _____ Date: _____

Skill:

Steps	Completed	Comments

Self-assessment	Evaluation/ validation methods	Levels	Type of validation	Comments
❏ Experienced ❏ Need practice ❏ Never done ❏ Not applicable (based on scope of practice)	❏ Verbal ❏ Demonstration/ observation ❏ Practical exercise ❏ Interactive class	❏ Beginner ❏ Intermediate ❏ Expert	❏ Orientation ❏ Annual ❏ Other _____	

_____   _____
Employee signature   *Observer signature*

FIGURE 6.2

RN Competency-Based Orientation Checklist

RN SKILLS ASSESSMENT/EVALUATION

NAME: _____ HIRE DATE: _____
UNIT: _____

STAFF DEVELOPMENT: INITIALS: PRECEPTORS: INITIALS:

_____   _____   _____   _____

_____   _____   _____   _____

_____   _____   _____   _____

Directions:

Orientee: Complete the self-assessment by placing a check (✓) in the appropriate column based on your level of familiarity or experience with each competency.

Staff Development/Preceptor: Complete the evaluation section for each competency after the orientee has demonstrated successful completion of that competency. Place the date and your initials in the appropriate column. If NE (not evaluated) is checked, include an explanation in the comments column.

Competencies	SELF-ASSESSMENT			EVALUATION			
	Comfortable	Need review	Have never done	* SD ORT	Unit	**NE	Comments
I. Competency A. Applies a systematic problem-solving approach in the implementation of nursing plans of care:							
1. Uses nursing process to systematically assess, plan, implement, and evaluate nursing care							

*SD ORT = Staff Development Orientation **NE = If Not Evaluated, indicate explanation

        Competency Management in Long-Term Care

FIGURE 6.2 (CONT.)

RN Competency-Based Orientation Checklist

Competencies	SELF-ASSESSMENT			EVALUATION			
	Comfortable	Need review	Have never done	* SD ORT	Unit	**NE	Comments
2. Provide/documents patient teaching/ discharge planning							
3. Involves patient/ significant other in plan of care							
4. Prioritizes nursing care for a group of patients							
5. Initiates patient referrals as needed							
6. Utilizes appropriate resources							
B. **Medication administration**							
1. Describes usual dose, common side effects, compatibilities, action, and untoward reactions of medications.							
2. Administers medications							
a. I.M.							
b. SQ and Insulin							
c. Calculations							
d. Other							
3. Documents administra- tion of medications (MAR, controlled drugs, etc.)							
4. Identifies medication error reporting system							

*SD ORT = Staff Development Orientation **NE = If Not Evaluated, indicate explanation

FIGURE 6.2 (CONT.)

RN Competency-Based Orientation Checklist

Competencies	SELF-ASSESSMENT			EVALUATION			
	Comfortable	Need review	Have never done	* SD ORT	Unit	**NE	Comments
C. Treatment and procedures							
1. Maintains gastric feeding tubes							
2. Inserts and maintains urinary catheters							
3. Performs trach care and suctioning							
4. Assesses patient safety, including proper utilization of restraints							
5. Incorporates nursing measures to reduce and prevent the spread of infection in daily nursing care							
6. Completes American Heart Association CPR guidelines							
7. Changes oxygen gauge and sets rate							
8. Locates various items on the emergency cart							
9. Identifies nursing responsibilities in emergency situations							
10. Completes: a. Admission of a patient							
b. Transfer of a patient							
c. Discharge of a patient							
11. Performs neurological checks when appropriate							
12. Other							

*SD ORT = Staff Development Orientation **NE = If Not Evaluated, indicate explanation

FIGURE 6.2 (CONT.)

RN Competency-Based Orientation Checklist

Competencies	SELF-ASSESSMENT			EVALUATION			
	Comfortable	Need review	Have never done	* SD ORT	Unit	**NE	Comments
II. Communication							
A. Documents on the following forms:							
• Initial Interdisciplinary Assessment							
• Nursing Discharge/ Patient Teaching							
• Interdisciplinary Plan of Care							
• Unusual Occurrence							
B. Transcribes physician's orders							
C. Takes verbal orders from physician							
D. Uses correct lines of communication							
E. Gives prompt, accurate, and pertinent shift report							
F. Interacts with patients, significant others, and health team members in positive manner							

*SD ORT = Staff Development Orientation **NE = If Not Evaluated, indicate explanation

© 2009 HCPro, Inc.

FIGURE 6.2 (CONT.)

RN Competency-Based Orientation Checklist

Competencies	SELF-ASSESSMENT			EVALUATION			
	Comfortable	Need review	Have never done	* SD ORT	Unit	**NE	Comments
III. Accountability/ Leadership							
A. Delegates patient care to other personnel appropriately							
B. Follows appropriate employee policies and procedures (i.e. call off, time off, LOA, etc.)							
C. Conforms to dress code							
D. Identifies role of the nurse in quality assurance							
E. Maintains safe working environment							
F. Contains costs through proper use of supplies and maintenance of equipment							
IV. Other							

*SD ORT = Staff Development Orientation **NE = If Not Evaluated, indicate explanation

Source: Summa Health System Hospitals, Akron, OH Reprinted with permission.

FIGURE 6.3

CNA Competency-Based Orientation Checklist

CNA Skills Assessment/Evaluation

NAME: _____ HIRE DATE: _____

UNIT: _____

STAFF DEVELOPMENT: INITIALS: PRECEPTORS: INITIALS:

_____ _____ _____ _____

_____ _____ _____ _____

_____ _____ _____ _____

Directions:

Orientee: Complete the self-assessment by placing a check (✓) in the appropriate column based on your level of familiarity or experience with each competency.

Staff Development/Preceptor: Complete the evaluation section for each competency after the orientee has demonstrated successful completion of that competency. Place the date and your initials in the appropriate column. If NE (not evaluated) is checked, include an explanation in the comments column.

	SELF-ASSESSMENT			EVALUATION			
Competencies	Comfortable	Need review	Have never done	* SD ORT	Unit	**NE	Comments
A. Demonstrates ability to do basic patient care as follows:							
1. Complete bed bath							
2. Partial bath							
3. Assists with shower							
4. Oral hygiene							
5. Back care							
6. Peri care							
7. Hair care							

*SD ORT = Staff Development Orientation **NE = If Not Evaluated, indicate explanation

FIGURE 6.3 (CONT.)

CNA Competency-Based Orientation Checklist

Competencies	SELF-ASSESSMENT			EVALUATION			
	Comfortable	Need review	Have never done	* SD ORT	Unit	**NE	Comments
8. Offering/removal of bed pan/urinal							
9. Cath care							
10. Documentation of output on Kardex or worksheet							Unit-based competency on file.
11. Feeding of patient, including compensatory strategies for feeding dysphagic patient							
12. Shaving of patient							
13. Occupied bed							
14. Unoccupied bed							
15. Accurately measuring patient intake and output and recording on appropriate form							
16. Patient transfer/ discharge							
B. Body mechanics							
1. Discusses the proper techniques of lifting/ turning/transferring patient							
2. Demonstrates proper technique in transferring patient from bed to cart and back							
3. Demonstrates proper technique transferring patient from bed to wheelchair							
4. Demonstrates proper technique in positioning and turning patients							

*SD ORT = Staff Development Orientation **NE = If Not Evaluated, indicate explanation

 Competency Management in Long-Term Care

FIGURE 6.3 (CONT.)

CNA Competency-Based Orientation Checklist

Competencies	SELF-ASSESSMENT			EVALUATION			
	Comfortable	Need review	Have never done	* SD ORT	Unit	**NE	Comments
C. Technical skills							
1. Assesses patient safety, including proper utilization and documentation of restraints							
2. Identifies responsibilities in emergency situations							
3. Incorporates measures to reduce and prevent the spread of infection in daily patient care							
D. Demonstrates ability to take and record vital signs.							Unit-based competency checklist on file
1. Temperature: • Takes oral temperature and records • Discusses procedure for rectal temperature							
2. Radial pulse: • Counts and records pulse rate							
3. Respirations: • Counts respiratory rate and records							
E. Demonstrates ability to obtain and transport appropriately the following specimens:							
1. Urine/routine/ccms							
2. Stool							

*SD ORT = Staff Development Orientation **NE = If Not Evaluated, indicate explanation

FIGURE 6.3 (CONT.)

CNA Competency-Based Orientation Checklist

Competencies	SELF-ASSESSMENT			EVALUATION			
	Comfortable	Need review	Have never done	* SD ORT	Unit	**NE	Comments
F. Performs postmortem care							
G. Removes dirty linen or equipment from patient room							
H. Passes and picks up trays							
1. Records intake (and output) accurately on worksheet in room							Unit-based competency checklist on file
2. Empty and replace trash bags, remove excess linen, etc., from patient rooms							
I. Maintenance needs							
1. Verbalizes safety issues with equipment (step ladders, hand tools, light bulbs, etc.)							
2. Identifies light maintenance duties							
J. Demonstrates proper use of communication							Unit-based competency checklist on file
1. Patient intercom							
2. Answering patient call light							

*SD ORT = Staff Development Orientation **NE = If Not Evaluated, indicate explanation

FIGURE 6.3 (CONT.)

CNA Competency-Based Orientation Checklist

Competencies	SELF-ASSESSMENT			EVALUATION			
	Comfortable	Need review	Have never done	* SD ORT	Unit	**NE	Comments
3. Telephone/answering phone appropriately by identifying unit, name, and status							
4. Explaining the importance of resident confidentiality							
5. Communicating to RN any unusual observations (signs and symptoms)							
K. Interacts with resident, significant others, and health team members in positive manner							
L. Safety issues (Each orientee should be able to discuss and correctly answer questions on the following safety topics)							
1. Fire safety							
2. Bomb threat							
3. Infection prevention and exposure control							
4. Disaster							
5. Evacuation							
6. Back safety							
7. Severe weather							
8. Electrical safety							

*SD ORT = Staff Development Orientation **NE = If Not Evaluated, indicate explanation

---

FIGURE 6.3 (CONT.)

CNA Competency-Based Orientation Checklist

Competencies	SELF-ASSESSMENT			EVALUATION			
	Comfortable	Need review	Have never done	* SD ORT	Unit	**NE	Comments
M. Punctuality							
1. Arrives on unit in uniform on time							
2. Notifies nursing office of absence according to policy							
3. Notifies nursing office of lateness according to policy							
4. Notifies nurse in charge when leaving unit and reason							
5. Follows guidelines for breaks and lunch hours							
6. Returns from errands and meetings promptly							
N. Tests							

*SD ORT = Staff Development Orientation **NE = If Not Evaluated, indicate explanation

Source: Summa Health System Hospitals, Akron, OH Reprinted with permission.

FIGURE 6.4

Competencies Tracking Sheet

COMPETENCY CHECKLIST

UNIT: _____

EMPLOYEE NAME	1. Mandatory Safety Education	2. Heart Saver	See Schedule for Mandatory Ed. and SLPs	UNIT-BASED					

COMPETENCY VERIFIED

Source: Summa Health System Hospitals, Akron, OH. Reprinted with permission.

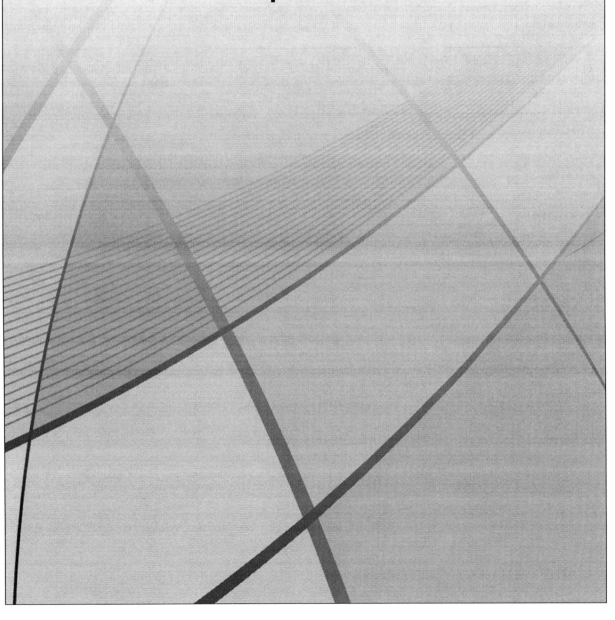

CHAPTER 7

Competencies

Competencies

Admission: Licensed Nurse 77

Admission: Nurse Assistant 78

Ambulation 79

Care of Resident with Aphasia 80

Bed Bath..81

Bed Making: Fully Occupied Bed...83

Bed Making: Fully Unoccupied Bed...85

Assisting with the Bedpan 86

Use of Bed Rails..87

Bladder Irrigation 88

Bladder Retraining and Toileting..89

Blood Pressure 90

Bowel Retraining 91

Call Lights 92

Care of Resident with Cancer...93

Catheter Care 94

Application of the External Catheter...95

Catheterization 97

Catheter Removal 102

Care of Resident Receiving Chemotherapy 103

Colostomy Care 104

Colostomy Irrigation 106

Denture Care 108

Care of Resident with Depression 109

Care of Resident with Diabetes...110

Care of Resident Receiving Dialysis Treatment..111

Anticipated Discharge..112

Discharge Against Medical Advice 114

Care of the Disoriented Resident 115

Clean Dressing Application 116

Sterile Dressing Application 117

Cleansing Enema 118

Prefilled Enema 119

Care of a Resident with Fragile Skin 120

Gait Belt 121

Gastrostomy Feedings 122

Gastrostomy Tube Insertions 123

Checking the Placement of a Gastrostomy Feeding Tube 124

Gastrostomy Tube Removal 125

Hearing Aid Care 126

Heimlich Maneuver 127

Mechanical Lift 128

Prefilled Oxygen Humidifiers 129

Intramuscular Injections 130

Subcutaneous Injections 131

Care of the Resident with Insomnia 132

Lab Result Reporting 133

Linen Handling 134

Medication Administration 135

Medication Errors 136

Missing Resident 137

Postmortem Care: Preparing the Body 140

Postmortem Care: Licensed Nurse 141

Nasogastric Tube Feedings 142

Nasogastric Tube Insertion 143

Checking the Placement of a Nasogastric Feeding Tube 144

Nasogastric Tube Removal 145

Oral Hygiene 146

Oral Hygiene for Unconscious Residents 147

Oxygen Administration 148

Pacemaker Checks 149

Psychotherapeutic Medication Use 150

Positioning 151

Taking a Pulse 152

Care of the Resident Receiving Radiation Treatments 153

Care of the Resident with Renal Disease 154

Range of Motion Exercises 155

Respirations 156

Care of the Resident with Respiratory Disease 157

Restraints 158

Seizure Precautions 159

Self-Determination and No CPR Requests 160

Self-Administration of Medications 161

Care of the Resident Who Has Public Displays of Sexual Behaviors 162

Shampoo 163

Shower 164

Arteriovenous Shunt Care 165

Monitoring the Side Effects for Psychosocial Medications 166

Sitz Bath 167

Foley Catheter Urine Specimen Collection 168

Mid-Stream Urine Specimen Collection 169

Routine Urine Specimen Collection 170

Sputum Specimen Collection 171

Stool Specimen Collection 172

Staple Removal 174

Suctioning 176

Rectal Suppository Administration 178

Vaginal Suppository Administration 179

Suture Removal 180

Syringe Feeding 182

TED Hose 184

Oral Temperature 185

Rectal Temperature 186

Transferring a Resident Out of the Facility 187

Serving Meals 188

Assisting with the Urinal 190

Vaginal Irrigation 191

Caring for the Wandering Resident 192

Weights 194

Assessing the Carotid Artery for a Bruit 195

Name: _____ Date: _____

Skill: **Admission: Licensed Nurse**

Steps	Completed	Comments
1. Introduce yourself to the resident and family. Ensure that the resident has been oriented.		
2. Assess for any immediate needs such as hunger, pain, or comfort.		
3. Screen the resident and perform a thorough body check. Complete the admission assessment form. Orient the resident to use of the call signal before leaving room.		
4. Call the attending physician and obtain admission orders.		
5. Notify the pharmacy, therapy, dietary, lab, or X-ray of orders, as appropriate.		
6. Take off orders for medications, treatments, and restorative, and record them on the appropriate sheets.		
7. Complete the telephone orders form.		
8. Initiate the care plan.		
9. Write an admission nurses note.		
10. Check the resident prior to leaving duty.		
11. Report the admission to the incoming nurse.		

Self-assessment	Evaluation/ validation methods	Levels	Type of validation	Comments
❏ Experienced ❏ Need practice ❏ Never done ❏ Not applicable (based on scope of practice)	❏ Verbal ❏ Demonstration/ observation ❏ Practical exercise ❏ Interactive class	❏ Beginner ❏ Intermediate ❏ Expert	❏ Orientation ❏ Annual ❏ Other _____	

_____
Employee signature

_____
Observer signature

Name: _____ Date: _____

Skill: **Admission: Nurse Assistant**

Steps	Completed	Comments
Prior to admission, check the room to ensure it is clean and in order. Bring permanent equipment to the room that will be needed for resident care.		
1. Introduce yourself to the resident and family.		
2. Assess for comfort (such as warmth, hunger, and pain). Report immediate needs to the charge nurse.		
3. Orient the resident and family to the call light and facility.		
4. Ask the resident or family whether they have any questions.		
5. Take the vital signs. Obtain the height and weight.		
6. Unpack clothes and complete the clothing list. Ensure that all items are labeled. If there are valuables, notify the charge nurse to ensure that they are recorded or stored appropriately. If there is an appliance, record identification number. Assist the resident to put items away, as needed.		
7. Ensure that the resident is comfortable and knows how to use the call signal before leaving the room.		

Self-assessment	Evaluation/ validation methods	Levels	Type of validation	Comments
❑ Experienced ❑ Need practice ❑ Never done ❑ Not applicable (based on scope of practice)	❑ Verbal ❑ Demonstration/ observation ❑ Practical exercise ❑ Interactive class	❑ Beginner ❑ Intermediate ❑ Expert	❑ Orientation ❑ Annual ❑ Other _____	

_____
Employee signature

_____
Observer signature

Name: _____   Date: _____

Skill: **Ambulation**

Steps	Completed	Comments
1. Explain the procedure to the resident and bring any assistive device, such as a walker or cane, to the bedside.		
2. Assist the resident with clothing and shoes appropriate to the floor surface, as needed.		
3. Stand the resident up slowly and wait until the resident is stably standing before attempting to ambulate.		
4. If using a gait belt, securely apply the gait belt around the resident's waist.		
5. If using a gait belt, walk along the side of the resident while maintaining a firm, underhand grasp in the center back of the belt.		
6. If the resident is unsteady, place one arm around the resident's waist and your other arm around the resident's upper arm. If the resident begins to fall, pull him or her close to your body. Ease the resident down your leg to the floor, while protecting the head.		
7. Encourage the resident to use the handrails if not using an assistive device.		
8. Stop and rest if the resident is tired.		
9. Stop ambulation if there is dizziness or pain and report it to the charge nurse.		

Self-assessment	Evaluation/ validation methods	Levels	Type of validation	Comments
❏ Experienced ❏ Need practice ❏ Never done ❏ Not applicable (based on scope of practice)	❏ Verbal ❏ Demonstration/ observation ❏ Practical exercise ❏ Interactive class	❏ Beginner ❏ Intermediate ❏ Expert	❏ Orientation ❏ Annual ❏ Other _____	

_____   _____
Employee signature   **Observer signature**

Name: _____ Date: _____

Skill: **Care of Resident with Aphasia**

Steps	Completed	Comments
1. Use short, simple words and sentences. Pronounce them clearly and slowly.		
2. Explain what will be done.		
3. Focus on one topic.		
4. Use gentle touch to show that you care.		
5. Keep the conversation short, but frequent.		
6. Use your facial expressions and gestures/body language to convey your message.		
7. Listen carefully to the response. Pay close attention to what the resident is saying.		
8. If you think you understand what the resident is saying, use paraphrasing to give the resident feedback.		
9. Allow the resident time to finish speaking. Don't cut him or her off.		
10. Monitor your body language. Avoid communicating frustration due to your inability to understand.		
11. Don't assume that the resident understands you if you are not sure and cannot get a response.		
12. Encourage the resident to point to things and use gestures.		
13. Use adaptive devices, such as picture boards, if available. The speech-language pathologist will often provide these devices and teach the resident to use them.		
14. Tell the resident when you are leaving the room. Make sure the resident is comfortable and safe, with the call signal and needed personal items within reach.		

Self-assessment	Evaluation/ validation methods	Levels	Type of validation	Comments
❑ Experienced ❑ Need practice ❑ Never done ❑ Not applicable (based on scope of practice)	❑ Verbal ❑ Demonstration/ observation ❑ Practical exercise ❑ Interactive class	❑ Beginner ❑ Intermediate ❑ Expert	❑ Orientation ❑ Annual ❑ Other _____	

_____   _____
Employee signature   **Observer signature**

Name: _____ Date: _____

Skill: **Bed Bath**

Steps	Completed	Comments
1. Explain the purpose and procedure to the resident.		
2. Assist with toileting, if needed.		
3. Get a basin with warm water and soap and clean towels and wash cloths.		
4. Pull the curtain. Drape the resident with a bath blanket for warmth, dignity, and modesty. Expose only the part of the body on which you are working.		
5. Encourage the resident to perform as much of the bath as possible.		
6. Fold the washcloth and wet with plain water. Do not add soap. Gently wash one eye from the inner corner out. Turn the cloth, and wash the other eye using a different part of cloth.		
7. Wet the washcloth and apply soap, according to the resident's preference. Wash, rinse, and pat dry face, neck, ears, and behind ears.		
8. Remove the resident's gown. Ensure that the resident is not exposed needlessly. Place a towel under the far arm.		
9. Wash, rinse, and pat dry the hand, arm, shoulder, and underarm.		
10. Move the towel and repeat with the near arm.		
11. Place a towel over the chest and abdomen. Lower the bath blanket to the waist. Lift the towel to wash, rinse, and dry the chest and abdomen, exposing only the area you are working on. Place a towel under the far leg. Wash, rinse, and pat the leg and foot dry.		
12. Repeat with the other leg and foot.		
13. Change the bath water.		
14. Turn the resident to the side.		
15. Wash, rinse, and dry from the neck to the buttocks, including the anal area.		

16. Change the water. Remove and discard gloves, if worn. Wash hands and obtain a new pair of gloves. Obtain a fresh washcloth and towel.		
17. Provide perineal care.		

Self-assessment	Evaluation/ validation methods	Levels	Type of validation	Comments
❏ Experienced ❏ Need practice ❏ Never done ❏ Not applicable (based on scope of practice)	❏ Verbal ❏ Demonstration/ observation ❏ Practical exercise ❏ Interactive class	❏ Beginner ❏ Intermediate ❏ Expert	❏ Orientation ❏ Annual ❏ Other _____	

Employee signature   **Observer signature**

                    Competency Management in Long-Term Care

| Name: _____ | Date: _____ |

Skill: **Bed Making: Fully Occupied Bed**

Steps	Completed	Comments
1. Explain the procedure to the resident.		
2. Place clean linen on overbed table, stacked in order of use.		
3. Lower the head of the bed.		
4. Drape the resident with a blanket, then pull top covers out from underneath while holding the bath blanket in place.		
5. Position the resident on his or her side, and ensure that side rail is up on the opposite side.		
6. Loosen the bottom linens and roll linen toward the resident, tucking it snugly against the resident's back.		
7. Fanfold the bottom sheet to the center of bed. If using a fitted sheet, fit the corners over the mattress. If using a flat sheet, miter the corner and tuck it in.		
8. Turn the resident onto his or her back, raise the side rail, move to the other side of the bed, and lower the side rail. Turn the resident away from you toward the side rail.		
9. Loosen the soiled linen, rolling linen from the head to foot of the bed. Discard the dirty linen in a plastic bag or place it in the soiled linen hamper in the hallway. Do not place on floor.		
10. Unroll and unfold the bottom bed linen. For a fitted sheet, fit it over corners of the bed. For a flat sheet, miter the corners.		
11. Position the resident in the supine position and raise the side rail.		
12. Remove the pillow and apply a clean pillowcase.		
13. Unfold the clean top sheet and place it over the blanket. Remove the blanket by pulling it out from underneath the sheet.		
14. Place the blanket over the sheet, and make a cuff by folding the top sheet over the blanket.		
15. Miter the corners and tuck in at the bottom, loosening the sheet around the resident's feet.		

16. Raise the side rail and repeat on the opposite side of the bed.		
17. Position the resident comfortably, with the call light and needed personal items within reach.		

Self-assessment	Evaluation/ validation methods	Levels	Type of validation	Comments
❏ Experienced ❏ Need practice ❏ Never done ❏ Not applicable (based on scope of practice)	❏ Verbal ❏ Demonstration/ observation ❏ Practical exercise ❏ Interactive class	❏ Beginner ❏ Intermediate ❏ Expert	❏ Orientation ❏ Annual ❏ Other _____	

_____
Employee signature

_____
Observer signature

Name: _____   Date: _____

Skill: **Bed Making: Fully Unoccupied Bed**

Steps	Completed	Comments
1. Explain the procedure to the resident.		
2. Stack clean linen on overbed table in order of use. If blanket or spread are to be reused, fold and place on bedside chair.		
3. Remove soiled linen by rolling it inward to avoid shaking. Check the linen for lost articles, such as dentures, glasses, and hearing aids. Discard linen in soiled linen hamper in hallway, or place in plastic bag or pillowcase until it can be removed from room. Do not place on floor.		
4. Place the bed flat at a comfortable height.		
5. Place the bottom sheet on the mattress with the sheet at the edge of the mattress by the foot end. Ensure that the sheet completely covers the mattress. Miter the corners and tuck in completely. Ensure that the sheet is tight.		
6. Fanfold the bottom sheet to the center of the bed and fit (fitted sheet) or miter (flat sheet) the corners.		
7. Fanfold the top sheet to the center of the bed.		
8. Fanfold the blanket over the top sheet.		
9. Place the bedspread over the bed, if used.		
10. Tuck the top linen under the foot of the mattress and miter the corner.		
11. Move to the other side of the bed.		
12. Fit the corners of the bottom sheet, unfold the top linen, tucking it under foot of the mattress, then miter the corner.		
13. Fold the top of the sheet over the blanket, forming a cuff.		
14. Put a clean pillowcase on the pillow. Place it at the head of the bed with the open end away from the door.		
15. Pull the bedspread down over the pillow and tuck the bedspread under lower edge of pillow.		

Self-assessment	Evaluation/ validation methods	Levels	Type of validation	Comments
❏ Experienced ❏ Need practice ❏ Never done ❏ Not applicable (based on scope of practice)	❏ Verbal ❏ Demonstration/ observation ❏ Practical exercise ❏ Interactive class	❏ Beginner ❏ Intermediate ❏ Expert	❏ Orientation ❏ Annual ❏ Other _____	

_____   _____
Employee signature   **Observer signature**

Name: _____ Date: _____

Skill: **Assisting with the Bedpan**

Steps	Completed	Comments
1. Explain the reason and procedure to the resident. Wash your hands. Apply gloves!		
2. Screen the resident. Lower the head of the bed.		

3. A. If the resident is able to lift his or her buttocks up:
   • Ask the resident to lift the hips and slip the bedpan under him or her.
   • Roll the head of the bed up slightly (30 to 45 degrees)
   • Place the toilet tissue near the resident
   • Place the call light near the resident
 	
  B. If the resident is unable to lift him or herself up:
   • Roll the resident on his or her side facing away from you. Place the bedpan. Hold it in place while rolling the resident back into the supine position.
   • Roll the head of the bed up slightly (30 to 45 degrees).
   • Place the toilet tissue near the resident.
   • Place the call light near the resident.		

4. Check on the resident frequently and remove the bedpan when finished.		
5. Assist the resident in using the toilet tissue being careful to wipe from front to back on female residents.		
6. Assist the resident in washing his or her hands.		
7. Position for comfort.		
8. Empty and disinfect the bedpan.		
9. Return the bedpan to the bedside cabinet, ensuring that it is not in contact with personal care items.		
10. Wash your hands.		

Self-assessment	Evaluation/ validation methods	Levels	Type of validation	Comments

❏ Experienced
❏ Need practice
❏ Never done
❏ Not applicable
   (based on scope
   of practice)
	❏ Verbal
	❏ Demonstration/
	   observation
	❏ Practical exercise
	❏ Interactive class
		❏ Beginner
		❏ Intermediate
		❏ Expert
			❏ Orientation
			❏ Annual
			❏ Other
			   _____	

_____   _____

Employee signature   **Observer signature**

Name: _____ Date: _____

Skill: **Use of Bed Rails**

Steps	Completed	Comments
1. Explain the purpose of bed rails to the resident or family.		
2. Explain the complications or risks of bed rails to the resident or family.		
3. If the resident or family wish bed rails to be used, complete a bed rail assessment and attempt less restrictive measures such as pillows, bolsters, or body pillows. Contact the physician for an order. If the resident is not capable of making a decision and the family or responsible party is unavailable, complete an interdisciplinary bed rail assessment and discuss the results with the physician. Obtain a physician order and signed release for their use.		
4. Monitor residents who use bed rails at least every two hours (or more often, if indicated) to ensure that the rails are up and the resident is safe. The call signal and needed personal items must be in reach.		

Self-assessment	Evaluation/ validation methods	Levels	Type of validation	Comments
❏ Experienced ❏ Need practice ❏ Never done ❏ Not applicable (based on scope of practice)	❏ Verbal ❏ Demonstration/ observation ❏ Practical exercise ❏ Interactive class	❏ Beginner ❏ Intermediate ❏ Expert	❏ Orientation ❏ Annual ❏ Other _____	

_____
Employee signature

_____
Observer signature

Name: _____ Date: _____

Skill: **Bladder Irrigation**

Steps	Completed	Comments
1. Explain the reason and procedure to the resident.		
2. Wash your hands.		
3. Bring the supplies needed to the bed side and screen the resident.		
4. Apply gloves.		
5. Wipe the junction of the catheter and connecting tubing before disconnecting.		
6. Using sterile technique, disconnect the catheter and place the tip in the sterile tray.		
7. Wipe the tip of the catheter with disinfecting solution and insert the tip of the irrigation syringe.		
8. Slowly depress the plunger, or squeeze the bulb, depending on type of syringe used. Never force the solution.		
9. Place the catheter tip in the sterile tray and allow the solution to drain out. If necessary, refill the syringe and repeat until the prescribed amount of irrigating solution has been instilled.		
10. Wipe the end of the catheter and drainage tube with an alcohol sponge. Allow the alcohol to dry before reattaching the drainage tubing to the catheter.		
11. Remove your gloves.		
12. Position the resident comfortably with the call light available.		
13. Wash your hands.		
14. Chart the results.		

Self-assessment	Evaluation/ validation methods	Levels	Type of validation	Comments
❏ Experienced ❏ Need practice ❏ Never done ❏ Not applicable (based on scope of practice)	❏ Verbal ❏ Demonstration/ observation ❏ Practical exercise ❏ Interactive class	❏ Beginner ❏ Intermediate ❏ Expert	❏ Orientation ❏ Annual ❏ Other _____	

_____
Employee signature

_____
Observer signature

Name: _____ Date: _____

Skill: **Bladder Retraining and Toileting**

Steps	Completed	Comments
1. Assess the resident to ensure he or she is capable of retraining and will cooperate with the retraining.		
2. Fill out the bladder retraining document. Circle times to be assessed and write any additional instructions. This will serve as a baseline to tell you when the resident is usually incontinent.		
3. Care plan the retraining.		
4. Assess the bladder incontinence for one week to determine whether there is a pattern for incontinence.		
5. Praise positive results. Give encouragement if there is an incontinent episode.		
6. Explain all procedures and the reasons for the procedures prior to performing them.		
7. Evaluate the progress each week and individualize the program by changing the times. Note any patterns of incontinence and schedule toileting or bedpans one hour prior.		
8. If there is no progress, reassess method and timing of training. If the resident appears not to benefit from the program after two weeks, discontinue the program.		
9. Update the bladder assessment and care plan when the program is discontinued.		

Self-assessment	Evaluation/ validation methods	Levels	Type of validation	Comments
❏ Experienced ❏ Need practice ❏ Never done ❏ Not applicable (based on scope of practice)	❏ Verbal ❏ Demonstration/ observation ❏ Practical exercise ❏ Interactive class	❏ Beginner ❏ Intermediate ❏ Expert	❏ Orientation ❏ Annual ❏ Other _____	

_____   _____
Employee signature   **Observer signature**

Name: _____ Date: _____

Skill: **Blood Pressure**

Steps	Completed	Comments
1. Explain the procedure to the resident. Make sure the cuff fits the resident's arm. The length of the bladder should be 80% of the arm circumference.		
2. Apply the blood pressure cuff by wrapping it around the resident's arm, 1 inch above the ante-cubital space. The center of the bladder should be positioned over the medial aspect of the arm.		
3. Extend the arm and palpate for a brachial pulse.		
4. Clean the ear plugs with an alcohol wipe and place the stethoscope over the pulse.		
5. Inflate the cuff to 140 systolic.		
6. Slowly release the air by turning the valve on the bulb.		
7. Listen for a sound. When you hear it, note the closest number on the gauge. This is the systolic pressure.		
8. Continue listening until the pitch of the sound changes or the sound stops. Note the closest number on the gauge. This is the diastolic pressure. Continue to listen for 10 to 20 mm Hg below this sound.		
9. Open the screw completely and deflate the cuff.		
10. Remove the cuff.		
11. Record the reading and the time in the chart.		

Self-assessment	Evaluation/ validation methods	Levels	Type of validation	Comments
❏ Experienced ❏ Need practice ❏ Never done ❏ Not applicable (based on scope of practice)	❏ Verbal ❏ Demonstration/ observation ❏ Practical exercise ❏ Interactive class	❏ Beginner ❏ Intermediate ❏ Expert	❏ Orientation ❏ Annual ❏ Other _____	

_____   _____
Employee signature   **Observer signature**

Name: _____ Date: _____

Skill: **Bowel Retraining**

Steps	Completed	Comments
1. Assess the resident to ensure he or she is capable of retraining and will cooperate with retraining.		
2. Fill out bowel retraining document. Circle the times to be assessed and write any additional instructions.		
3. Care plan the retraining.		
4. Assess the bowel incontinence for one week to determine whether there is a pattern for incontinence.		
5. Follow the physician's orders for suppository use.		
6. Praise positive results.		
7. Explain all procedures and the reasons to the resident prior to performing them.		
8. Give the resident encouragement if there is an incontinent episode.		
9. Evaluate the progress each week and individualize the program. Note any patterns of incontinence and schedule toileting or bedpans one hour prior.		
10. If there is no progress for a two week period, reassess method and timing of training. If the resident appears not to benefit from the program, discontinue the program.		
11. Update the bowel assessment and care plan when program is discontinued.		

Self-assessment	Evaluation/ validation methods	Levels	Type of validation	Comments
❑ Experienced ❑ Need practice ❑ Never done ❑ Not applicable (based on scope of practice)	❑ Verbal ❑ Demonstration/ observation ❑ Practical exercise ❑ Interactive class	❑ Beginner ❑ Intermediate ❑ Expert	❑ Orientation ❑ Annual ❑ Other _____	

_____
Employee signature

_____
Observer signature

Name: _____ Date: _____

Skill: **Call Lights**

Steps	Completed	Comments
1. Explain the reason and functioning of the call light to the resident.		
2. Ensure that all residents (even those who are confused) have access to the call signal at all times and know how to use it. Obtain a hand bell if the resident cannot use the regular signal cord.		
3. All staff members are responsible for answering call signals, even for residents who are not part of their assignment. Know the various signals for resident rooms, bathrooms, etc. In general, a regular signal should be answered within 3 minutes and an emergency signal within 1 minute.		
4. Turn the signal off when you arrive.		
5. Respond to the resident's signal in an appropriate manner by asking how you may help.		
6. Monitor the lights and answer them promptly. Ensure that all lights are answered in a timely manner, such as within _____ minutes for a regular call signal and _____ minutes for an emergency signal. If an emergency occurs when you are in a resident's room, remain in the room and assist according to the limits of your job description and qualifications. Pull the emergency call signal; if possible, call out for help, or use the telephone, if available.		

Self-assessment	Evaluation/ validation methods	Levels	Type of validation	Comments
❏ Experienced ❏ Need practice ❏ Never done ❏ Not applicable (based on scope of practice)	❏ Verbal ❏ Demonstration/ observation ❏ Practical exercise ❏ Interactive class	❏ Beginner ❏ Intermediate ❏ Expert	❏ Orientation ❏ Annual ❏ Other _____	

_____
Employee signature

_____
Observer signature

Name:			Date:	

Skill: **Care of Resident with Cancer**

Steps	Completed	Comments
1. Monitor for weakness or tiredness and encourage naps, as needed.		
2. Assess the resident regularly for pain or other expected complications, such as nausea, and medicate when needed. Review the WHO pain ladder when considering medication dosages and combinations.		
3. Administer medication and lab work as ordered. Report abnormal results promptly.		
4. Encourage activities of choice.		
5. Report excessive weakness, pain, weight loss, sadness, poor appetite, or tiredness to physician.		
6. Encourage 80–100% of the diet.		
7. Monitor the weights and appetite.		
8. Encourage the resident to verbalize feelings and concerns over disease and attempt to resolve concerns. The resident and family will be in various steps of the grieving process. Understand their concerns and provide support.		
9. Allow the family to participate in care, if desired and as appropriate, considering the resident's wishes.		

Self-assessment	Evaluation/ validation methods	Levels	Type of validation	Comments
❏ Experienced ❏ Need practice ❏ Never done ❏ Not applicable (based on scope of practice)	❏ Verbal ❏ Demonstration/ observation ❏ Practical exercise ❏ Interactive class	❏ Beginner ❏ Intermediate ❏ Expert	❏ Orientation ❏ Annual ❏ Other _____	

_____
Employee signature

_____
Observer signature

Name: _____ Date: _____

Skill: **Catheter Care**

Steps	Completed	Comments
1. Explain the reason and procedure to the resident.		
2. Wash your hands and pull the curtain.		
3. Using clean warm water and a soapy washcloth, gently wash around the urinary meatus and catheter.		
4. Wet washcloth and apply soap or perineal cleaner sparingly to avoid irritation.		
5. First separate inner labia and wash down the center over the urethral area, wiping downward from front toward back and stopping at the base of labia.		
6. Continue to wash the rest of the perineal area, wiping from front to back, alternating from side to side and moving outward to the thighs.		
7. Then rinse well and dry the urethral and perineal area, working in the same direction until entire area is clean, soap-free, and dry.		

8. If indwelling urinary catheter is present:
• Hold catheter tubing to one side and support against leg to avoid traction or unnecessary movement of the catheter while washing perineum. Keep drainage bag below level of bladder.
• When washing, rinsing, and drying the urethral area:
  – Gently wash, rinse, and dry around the juncture of the catheter and meatus.
  – Wash the catheter from the meatus down the tube about 3 inches.		

Monitor for redness or pain.		
Rinse and gently pat dry.		
Position the bed linen and the resident.		

Self-assessment	Evaluation/ validation methods	Levels	Type of validation	Comments
❏ Experienced ❏ Need practice ❏ Never done ❏ Not applicable (based on scope of practice)	❏ Verbal ❏ Demonstration/ observation ❏ Practical exercise ❏ Interactive class	❏ Beginner ❏ Intermediate ❏ Expert	❏ Orientation ❏ Annual ❏ Other _____	

_____ _____
Employee signature **Observer signature**

| Name: _____ | Date: _____ |

Skill: **Application of the External Catheter**

Steps	Completed	Comments
1. Explain the reason and procedure to the resident.		
2. Wash your hands and put on gloves.		
3. If a sizing guide comes with the catheter: • Measure penis for appropriate external catheter size using the paper sizing guide • Wrap the sizing band around the penis immediately behind the glans • The end of the band with the black bar should be on the outside • Note the color and size where the black bar reaches • If the black bar is between two sizes, choose the larger size		
4. Gently clean the penis with soap and water and pat it dry with a towel. If a self-adhesive catheter is used, you may wish to trim pubic hair.		
5. Hold the penis straight and roll the condom portion over the penis. Leave at least a half inch of free catheter at the end of the penis to allow for drainage.		
6. Secure the condom loosely. An adhesive band is included in the packaging for most brands of catheters. If used, wrap in a spiral, and make sure it is not too tight. The band should never encircle the penis.		
7. Attach a catheter drainage bag or leg bag.		
8. Cover and position the resident.		
9. Remove your gloves.		
10. Wash your hands.		
11. Check the penis 5 to 10 minutes after application for evidence of constriction.		
12. Monitor for: • Cyanosis • Discoloration • Edema		

| 13. Observe the system every 4 hours. Check the appearance of the penis and urine flow. | | |
| 14. Remove the external catheter and wash and dry penis at least every 24 hours. | | |

Self-assessment	Evaluation/ validation methods	Levels	Type of validation	Comments
❏ Experienced ❏ Need practice ❏ Never done ❏ Not applicable (based on scope of practice)	❏ Verbal ❏ Demonstration/ observation ❏ Practical exercise ❏ Interactive class	❏ Beginner ❏ Intermediate ❏ Expert	❏ Orientation ❏ Annual ❏ Other _____	

Employee signature

Observer signature

Name: _____ Date: _____

Skill: **Catheterization**

Steps	Completed	Comments
1. Explain the reason and procedure to the resident.		
2. Wash your hands.		
3. Assist resident to lie on the back in the dorsal recumbant or lithotomy position, with knees bent and separated. If the resident cannot maintain this position due to discomfort, try flexing one knee and keeping the other leg flat on the bed. The female resident may be positioned in the Sims' position, if necessary.		
4. Place an underpad beneath the resident's buttocks. You may wish to use a facility underpad, then cover with the sterile pad from the catheter tray. (The sterile pad is not absorbent enough to contain spills.)		
5. Provide perineal care.		
6. Discard used supplies.		
7. Wash your hands.		
8. Clean and disinfect the overbed table. Cover the table with a drape, such as a towel or underpad if this is your preference or facility policy.		
9. Open the sterile catheterization tray and establish a sterile field.		
10. Open the catheter of the proper diameter and balloon size and drop it on the sterile field.		
11. Open a plastic trash bag and roll the top down slightly so it stays open. Place the bag at the foot of the bed, or a convenient location to contain trash and discarded supplies. *Position the bag so that you do not have to reach or cross over sterile supplies to discard soiled items.*		
12. Open the sterile pack and place the underpad beneath the resident.		
13. Pick up the first drape. Stand away from the bed and hold the drape away from your body, allowing it to unfold.		
14. Pick up the next drape. Stand away from the bed and allow the drape to unfold away from your body. Position it on the resident.		
15. Apply sterile gloves before obtaining the last drape.		

16. Pick up the fenestrated drape with your gloved hands and allow it to unfold. Center the opening in the drape over the perineum. If you must lift the penis to position the drape, use your nondominant hand. (This hand will be contaminated and cannot be used to contact sterile supplies.)		
17. Open the remaining packages in the tray and arrange items on the sterile field for your convenience.		
18. If no specimen will be collected, attach the indwelling catheter to the drainage bag.		
19. Close the clamp over the drainage spout.		
20. Attach the saline-filled syringe to the inflation port on the catheter. Test the balloon by injecting the fluid while checking the balloon for leaks. If the balloon leaks or will not inflate, replace the catheter.		
21. Pull back on the plunger of the syringe to deflate the balloon.		
22. Open the package of povidone-iodine or antiseptic solution. Open the cotton balls or applicators, if necessary. Pour the solution over the cotton balls or applicators.		
23. Open the package of water-soluble lubricant. Squeeze the lubricant onto a corner or side of the sterile packing tray.		
24. Lubricate the tip of the catheter for approximately 2 inches for a female and 4 to 5 inches for a male.		
25. Pick up the forceps in the tray. Using the forceps, grasp a moistened cotton ball.		
26. **_Female resident:_** • Separate the labia with the nondominant hand. Once you touch the skin, this glove is contaminated. • Keep the labia spread apart until the catheter has been inserted. If your hand accidentally slips, you must begin the cleansing procedure again if the sides of the labia contact each other. • Beginning in the center, wipe the labia from top to bottom, using a single stroke. Discard the cotton ball. • Pick up a second cotton ball and repeat the procedure on the side opposite where you are standing. Discard the cotton ball. • Pick up another cotton ball, and cleanse the labia closest to you from top to bottom. Discard the cotton ball. • If cotton remains after you have cleansed the labia using the sequence above, you may use the remaining cotton balls to pat the area dry. When you have finished, discard the cotton ball and forceps.		

27. **Male resident:** • Pick up the penis with the nondominant hand. Your glove is now contaminated. • Retract the foreskin. • Beginning at the urinary meatus, wipe the penis in a circular motion. Discard the cotton ball. • Pick up a second cotton ball and repeat, cleansing outward from the meatus in a circle. Discard the cotton ball. • Pick up a third cotton ball. Cleanse in another circle beyond the second circle, extending outward. At this point, you should have cleansed a large area. • If cotton remains after you have cleansed the penis using the sequence above, you may use the remaining cotton balls to pat the area dry. When you have finished, discard the cotton ball and forceps.		
28. If a specimen will be collected, remove the lid from the specimen cup. Position the open end of the catheter into the specimen collection container. (You may also use a drainage basin positioned in front of the resident.)		
29. With your dominant hand, pick up the catheter. Hold it approximately 1 ½ to 2 inches from the tip.		
30. Insert the catheter into the urethra.		
31. **Female resident:** • Visualize the urinary meatus. Inform the resident when you will be inserting the catheter. Instructing the resident to cough, bear down, or whistle will distract her and helps relax the urinary sphincter. • Insert the catheter through the external meatus and into the urethra, threading it into the bladder (about 1 ½ to 3 inches). • Hold the catheter in place without inflating the balloon until urine flows. If urine flow does not begin immediately, hold the catheter in place for a few minutes. • If no urine drains, the catheter may be in the vagina. *Leave it in place.* You must get fresh supplies and repeat the procedure. Leaving the original catheter in place will make it easier to find the urethra on the next attempt. • Remove it after the procedure is successful. If an assistant is helping you, continue to hold the labia apart, and send him or her for another catheter. When he or she returns, have the assistant open the catheter. Grasp it with your sterile hand, and repeat the insertion part of the procedure.		

32. **Male resident:** • Hold the penis upright with your nondominant hand. • Inform the resident when you will be inserting the catheter. Insert the catheter through the external meatus. • Instruct the resident to cough, bear down, or whistle while you are inserting the catheter. Encourage him to continue throughout the remainder of the procedure (until the catheter is in the bladder). • Advance the catheter until urine flows. • *Never force the catheter. If you meet resistance and are unable to advance the catheter, change the angle of the penis slightly (lower it to about 60 degrees), and try again. If you are still unsuccessful, lower the penis slightly again and try to advance the catheter. If you cannot advance the catheter beyond the prostate, do not force it. Stop the procedure and notify the physician of the problem.*		
33. Collect a specimen, if needed. Thirty to 50 mL of urine is necessary. After this amount has been collected, pinch the catheter to stop the flow of urine. Move the cup to the side and position the drainage basin under the end of the catheter. Allow the bladder to empty into the basin. If urine continues to flow after 1,000 mL of urine drains into the basin, pinch the catheter. Wait for 15 to 30 minutes and open the clamp. Allow the bladder to empty in 250 mL increments until empty. (Some facilities allow the bladder to empty completely on the first try. Know and follow your facility policy. This is a controversial area requiring further research.)		
34. Attach the syringe to the inflation port. Slowly push the plunger to inflate the balloon. Note how much fluid you instilled into the balloon and document this when you have finished the procedure.		
35. Attach the collection bag to the catheter, if this was not done previously.		
36. Replace the foreskin in the male resident.		
37. Hang the collection bag on the bed frame. Do not hang it from the siderails, and avoid letting it touch the floor.		

38. Tape the catheter or apply a Velcro leg strap. Never leave the room until the catheter is secured. The mechanical irritation caused by catheter movement can cause urethral and meatal tearing, accidental removal, and serious complications. For the female resident, secure the catheter to the upper thigh. The catheter in the male is secured to either the upper thigh (with a leg strap) or the abdomen (with tape).		
39. Remove the drapes. Tear the center of the fenestrated drape to remove it. Discard in the plastic bag.		
40. Initiate intake and output monitoring and place an I&O worksheet at the bedside.		
41. Position the resident for comfort and safety with the call signal and needed personal items within reach.		
42. Wash your hands.		
43. Discard trash from the procedure in the biohazardous waste when you leave the room.		
44. Document the procedure.		

Self-assessment	Evaluation/ validation methods	Levels	Type of validation	Comments
❏ Experienced ❏ Need practice ❏ Never done ❏ Not applicable (based on scope of practice)	❏ Verbal ❏ Demonstration/ observation ❏ Practical exercise ❏ Interactive class	❏ Beginner ❏ Intermediate ❏ Expert	❏ Orientation ❏ Annual ❏ Other _____	

_____
Employee signature

_____
Observer signature

Name: _____ Date: _____

Skill: **Catheter Removal**

Steps	Completed	Comments
1. Explain the reason and procedure to the resident.		
2. Wash your hands and pull the curtain. Put on your gloves.		
3. Position the resident on back with knees spread apart.		
4. Drape the resident.		
5. Place an incontinent pad under the buttocks.		
6. Remove the tape or Velcro strap securing the catheter to the resident's body.		
7. Withdraw the water from the balloon with a syringe. Monitor the amount removed to ensure that all the water is removed.		
8. Gently remove the catheter.		
9. Remove your gloves.		
10. Position the resident for comfort.		
11. Discard the catheter according to facility policy.		
12. Empty the urine drainage bag, measure and record the output, and discard the bag in the appropriate container.		
13. Continue to monitor intake and output to evaluate elimination pattern.		
14. When the resident voids, evaluate elimination for amount, appearance, odor, color, and clarity. Assess the bladder for potential urinary retention.		
15. Wash your hands.		
16. Evaluate the resident's ability to void. If he or she has not voided in 4 hours or complains of inability to void, assess the bladder and take the appropriate nursing action.		

Self-assessment	Evaluation/ validation methods	Levels	Type of validation	Comments
❏ Experienced ❏ Need practice ❏ Never done ❏ Not applicable (based on scope of practice)	❏ Verbal ❏ Demonstration/ observation ❏ Practical exercise ❏ Interactive class	❏ Beginner ❏ Intermediate ❏ Expert	❏ Orientation ❏ Annual ❏ Other _____	

_____ _____
Employee signature **Observer signature**

  Competency Management in Long-Term Care

Name: _____ Date: _____

Skill: **Care of Resident Receiving Chemotherapy**

Steps	Completed	Comments
1. Encourage rest after chemotherapy.		
2. Administer lab and medications as ordered with abnormals reported promptly.		
3. Notify the physician if nausea or vomiting occurs.		
4. Staff to monitor medications, diet, environment, and labs for possible complications.		
5. Encourage fluids.		
6. Assess resident for pain regularly. Give medication for discomfort if ordered. Evaluate and document response to medication. Report to the physician if ineffective.		
7. Visit with the resident when ill to help relieve anxiety.		
8. Monitor the diet for tolerance.		

Self-assessment	Evaluation/ validation methods	Levels	Type of validation	Comments
❑ Experienced ❑ Need practice ❑ Never done ❑ Not applicable (based on scope of practice)	❑ Verbal ❑ Demonstration/ observation ❑ Practical exercise ❑ Interactive class	❑ Beginner ❑ Intermediate ❑ Expert	❑ Orientation ❑ Annual ❑ Other _____	

_____
Employee signature

_____
Observer signature

Name: _____ Date: _____

Skill: **Colostomy Care**

Steps	Completed	Comments
1. Explain the reason and procedure to the resident.		
2. Wash your hands and pull the curtain.		
3. Put on your gloves.		
4. Position the bedpan near the resident, close to the stoma.		
5. Position the end of the appliance in the bedpan. Remove the clip at the bottom and empty into the bedpan.		
6. Gently lift the appliance to release the adhesive. Apply gentle traction on the skin with one hand while slowly lifting the pouch with the other.		
7. Remove the old colostomy bag and note drainage. Discard in plastic bag or put it to the side for cleaning and reuse, according to the type of device being used.		
8. Cleanse the stoma and surrounding tissue gently with warm water. Pat dry with a hand towel. If stool escapes, remove it with toilet tissue. Monitor the skin for changes in the size, color, or presence of redness or skin breakdown. Remember, this tissue is tender and fragile. Handle with care!		
9. Apply a barrier cream or prescribed product to the area surrounding the stoma.		
10. Change gloves, if soiled with stool.		
11. Check the opening in the new pouch to ensure that it is large enough to fit the diameter of the stoma. It should not fit tightly to the stoma, but should seal securely around the edges.		
12. Measure the stoma with a stoma measuring guide. (The flange wafer should be at least 1/2" larger than the stoma). Mark the paper backing.		
13. Enlarge the center hole of the wafer to the correct size.		
14. Check the size by gently placing the wafer over the stoma.		
15. Remove the paper backing from the wafer.		
16. Place a ring of stoma paste around the hole you've cut on the sticky side of the wafer.		
17. Apply skin prep to peristomal skin and allow to air dry.		

18. Hold the wafer by two side edges and position it with hole over the stoma.		
19. Place the ostomy bag over the stoma. Center the ring in the pouch over the stoma, with the large part of the pouch hanging down. Gently press it down over the skin with the palm of your hand.		
20. Make sure the adhesive is wrinklefree. Hold gentle pressure on the adhesive ring for a minute.		
21. If an ostomy belt is used, ensure that two fingers can be inserted beneath it to prevent pressure at stoma site.		
22. For added security, the wafer may be picture-framed with waterproof tape after using skin prep on the skin. (Avoid an alcohol-based skin prep.)		
23. Check the end of the pouch to ensure that it is closed and clamped securely.		
24. Remove your gloves.		
25. Position the resident for comfort and safety with the call signal and needed personal items within reach.		
26. Wash your hands.		
27. Chart the treatment.		

Self-assessment	Evaluation/ validation methods	Levels	Type of validation	Comments
❑ Experienced ❑ Need practice ❑ Never done ❑ Not applicable (based on scope of practice)	❑ Verbal ❑ Demonstration/ observation ❑ Practical exercise ❑ Interactive class	❑ Beginner ❑ Intermediate ❑ Expert	❑ Orientation ❑ Annual ❑ Other _____	

_____
Employee signature

_____
Observer signature

Name: _____   Date: _____

Skill: **Colostomy Irrigation**

Steps	Completed	Comments
1. Check the physician's orders and explain the reason and procedure to the resident.		
2. Wash your hands and screen the resident.		
3. Assist the resident to the bathroom if the procedure will be done there. If it will be done in bed, position an underpad to prevent soiling. Position a second underpad on a chair next to the bed, and place the bedpan on it.		
4. Hang the irrigation bag on an IV pole approximately 20 inches above the resident. The bottom of the bag should be at about the resident's shoulder level to prevent water from entering the bowel too rapidly.		
5. Prime the irrigation tubing, if this was not done previously.		
6. Put on your gloves.		
7. Turn the resident on the side of the colostomy and place the basin under the colostomy.		
8. Remove the colostomy bag and discard in a plastic bag or according to facility policy.		
9. Apply the irrigation sleeve, securing it with the adhesive backing or an appliance belt.		
10. Place the open end of the irrigation sleeve into the bedpan on a chair next to the bed (or in the toilet).		
11. If the procedure is done on the toilet, cut the bottom of the sleeve, if needed, so that it hangs slightly above water level. Avoid cutting it too short, as it may splash.		
12. Lubricate the small finger of your gloved hand.		
13. Insert the lubricated finger slowly and gently into the stoma. This will cause involuntary tightening of the stoma, but it will relax in a few minutes. Identify the angle of the bowel with your finger. You will insert the irrigation cone at this angle.		
14. Lubricate the cone on the irrigation set.		
15. Insert the cone gently and securely, in the direction of the bowel.		
16. Unclamp the tubing and allow the fluid to run in slowly. Adjust the flow with the roller clamp, or pinch the tubing, if necessary, to slow or control the flow rate.		
17. The fluid should run in over 10 to 15 minutes.		
18. Remove the cone when the bag is empty.		

19. If possible, remove the cone while water remains in the tubing, to avoid injecting air. Close the tip of the sleeve if the resident will be ambulating.		
20. Apply the colostomy bag.		
21. Remove your gloves and discard according to facility policy.		
22. If the resident will be ambulating, remove your gloves and wash your hands. Discard your gloves according to facility policy.		
23. If permitted by facility policy, and the resident is ambulatory, allow him or her to ambulate for 15 to 20 minutes until evacuation occurs. The ambulation will stimulate peristalsis in the bowel. Otherwise, the resident can remain stationary until elimination occurs. The nonambulatory resident can lean forward and massage the abdomen to stimulate peristalsis.		
24. When evacuation occurs, apply clean gloves.		
25. After the irrigation is complete, remove and discard the irrigation sleeve. If it is reusable, rinse it well and hang to air dry.		
26. Wash the skin surrounding the stoma with warm water. Pat dry. Apply barrier product, if ordered.		
27. Apply a clean appliance.		
28. Assist the resident with handwashing.		
29. Position the resident for comfort and safety with the call signal and needed personal items within reach.		
30. Wash your hands.		

Self-assessment	Evaluation/ validation methods	Levels	Type of validation	Comments
❏ Experienced ❏ Need practice ❏ Never done ❏ Not applicable (based on scope of practice)	❏ Verbal ❏ Demonstration/ observation ❏ Practical exercise ❏ Interactive class	❏ Beginner ❏ Intermediate ❏ Expert	❏ Orientation ❏ Annual ❏ Other _____	

_____   _____
Employee signature   **Observer signature**

Name: _____ Date: _____

Skill: **Denture Care**

Steps	Completed	Comments
1. Explain the reason and procedure to the resident.		
2. Wash your hands.		
3. At bedtime, remove the dentures and brush off the particles with a toothbrush.		
4. Place the dentures in a labeled denture cup with denture cleaning solution.		
5. Before breakfast, place the dentures in a basin and gently brush the particles off with a toothbrush.		
6. Rinse the dentures and insert them in the resident's mouth.		
7. Repeat the brushing during the day if the dentures become filled with particles.		
8. Wash your hands.		

Self-assessment	Evaluation/ validation methods	Levels	Type of validation	Comments
❑ Experienced ❑ Need practice ❑ Never done ❑ Not applicable (based on scope of practice)	❑ Verbal ❑ Demonstration/ observation ❑ Practical exercise ❑ Interactive class	❑ Beginner ❑ Intermediate ❑ Expert	❑ Orientation ❑ Annual ❑ Other _____	

_____ _____
Employee signature **Observer signature**

Name: _____ Date: _____

Skill: **Care of Resident with Depression**

Steps	Completed	Comments
1. Always approach the resident calmly and unhurriedly. Speak in a soothing voice.		
2. Encourage the resident to perform independent ADLs and decisions concerning the timing of care, clothes to wear, what activities to attend.		
3. LISTEN attentively.		
4. Allow resident to talk about the problem, if he or she wishes. Use silence to allow resident to think and continue talking (this shows respect and acceptance).		
5. Encourage and assist the resident to help staff in mutual problem solving of depression-causing stimuli.		
6. Encourage activities of the resident's choice and preference.		
7. Visit the resident in own room or other facility area for socialization and reinforcement of positive thoughts.		
8. Encourage the resident to discuss interests or concerns.		
9. Notify the physician if the behavior interferes with functioning.		
10. Monitor the weights, appetite, labs, and environment to assist the physician in determining the cause of depression.		

Self-assessment	Evaluation/ validation methods	Levels	Type of validation	Comments
❑ Experienced ❑ Need practice ❑ Never done ❑ Not applicable (based on scope of practice)	❑ Verbal ❑ Demonstration/ observation ❑ Practical exercise ❑ Interactive class	❑ Beginner ❑ Intermediate ❑ Expert	❑ Orientation ❑ Annual ❑ Other _____	

_____ _____
Employee signature   **Observer signature**

Name: _____ Date: _____

Skill: **Care of Resident with Diabetes**

Steps	Completed	Comments
1. Diet as ordered. Monitor intake.		
2. Administer medication and lab work as ordered. Report abnormal results promptly.		
3. Monitor for thirst, excessive appetite, or voiding, change in level of consciousness or mood, perspiring, and report to physician promptly.		
4. Special monitoring of skin for redness or circulatory problems.		
5. Monitor and ensure position changes.		
6. Encourage exercise and activity attendance.		

Self-assessment	Evaluation/ validation methods	Levels	Type of validation	Comments
❑ Experienced ❑ Need practice ❑ Never done ❑ Not applicable (based on scope of practice)	❑ Verbal ❑ Demonstration/ observation ❑ Practical exercise ❑ Interactive class	❑ Beginner ❑ Intermediate ❑ Expert	❑ Orientation ❑ Annual ❑ Other _____	

_____   _____
Employee signature   **Observer signature**

| Name: _____ | Date: _____ |

Skill: **Care of Resident Receiving Dialysis Treatment**

Steps	Completed	Comments
1. Monitor for signs of fluid overload secondary to little or no renal function: • Monitor feet and hands for edema. • Monitor for elevated blood pressure, shortness of breath, or chest pains. • Diet and Medications as ordered. *FLUID RESTRICTION as ordered. • Encourage the resident to be out of bed daily and exercise. • Monitor for nausea or vomiting.		
2. Monitor for hemorrhage secondary to heparin therapy during dialysis: • Monitor for bleeding from site, mouth, urine, or feces		
3. Monitor for infection or clotting of the access area. • Do not take the blood pressure in the arm with the dialysis access site • Monitor for swelling, pain, redness, or drainage of the shunt • Monitor bruit as ordered		
4. Administer special skin care to prevent itching.		
5. Arrange for dialysis, as ordered.		
6. Encourage the resident to attend activities daily.		
7. Practice good infection control and wear gloves when touching drainage, secretions, discharges, or dressings.		

Self-assessment	Evaluation/ validation methods	Levels	Type of validation	Comments
❑ Experienced ❑ Need practice ❑ Never done ❑ Not applicable (based on scope of practice)	❑ Verbal ❑ Demonstration/ observation ❑ Practical exercise ❑ Interactive class	❑ Beginner ❑ Intermediate ❑ Expert	❑ Orientation ❑ Annual ❑ Other _____	

_____
Employee signature

_____
Observer signature

Name: _____	Date: _____

Skill: **Anticipated Discharge**

Steps	Completed	Comments
1. Initiate discharge planning as soon as it is determined that discharge will occur.		
2. Discuss impending discharge with the resident.		
3. Communicate with the family regarding what, if any, referrals to agencies are needed. Contact agencies needed.		
4. Obtain a discharge order from the attending physician. Be sure to ascertain whether it is with or without medications.		
5. Complete the discharge summary. Nursing facilities are required to develop a postdischarge plan of care when the resident will be transferred to another facility, or to his or her own home. This requirement is the source of a great deal of confusion and many deficiencies on surveys. The requirement does not apply if the resident is transferred to the acute care hospital in an emergency and does not return to the facility.		
6. Pack and complete the clothing list.		
7. Assist the resident and family to arrange transportation.		
8. Ensure that the resident, family, or responsible party is given information concerning their right to appeal all discharges.		
9. Documentation: • When a resident leaves your care, document the time, the condition of the resident upon leaving, and any other information necessary to reflect the situation accurately. For example, if the resident is at risk for skin breakdown, document the complete condition of the skin. • When transferring a resident, state the date and time, resident condition, who accompanied the resident, who provided the transfer, where and to whom the resident is transferred, and manner of transfer (wheelchair, stretcher, ambulance, and so forth). Document the disposition of the resident's personal possessions and medications. List instructions given to the resident and teaching in anticipation of discharge.		

Self-assessment	Evaluation/ validation methods	Levels	Type of validation	Comments
❏ Experienced ❏ Need practice ❏ Never done ❏ Not applicable (based on scope of practice)	❏ Verbal ❏ Demonstration/ observation ❏ Practical exercise ❏ Interactive class	❏ Beginner ❏ Intermediate ❏ Expert	❏ Orientation ❏ Annual ❏ Other _____	

_____   _____
Employee signature   **Observer signature**

Name: _____ Date: _____

Skill: **Discharge Against Medical Advice**

Steps	Completed	Comments
1. Encourage the resident, family, or responsible party to discuss their motivation for wanting to leave the facility. Attempt to resolve their concerns.		
2. Inform the resident, family, or responsible party of the possible medical complications of their discharge action.		
3. Notify the attending physician.		
4. If unable to persuade them to stay, explain and have the Against Medical Advice form signed.		
5. Document incident in the nurses' notes, including any reasons given.		
6. Do NOT give medications.		

Self-assessment	Evaluation/ validation methods	Levels	Type of validation	Comments
❏ Experienced ❏ Need practice ❏ Never done ❏ Not applicable (based on scope of practice)	❏ Verbal ❏ Demonstration/ observation ❏ Practical exercise ❏ Interactive class	❏ Beginner ❏ Intermediate ❏ Expert	❏ Orientation ❏ Annual ❏ Other _____	

_____ _____
Employee signature **Observer signature**

Name: _____ Date: _____

Skill: Care of the Disoriented Resident

Steps	Completed	Comments
1. Explain all procedures. Use simple one word commands, if possible.		
2. Provide cuing and prompting for personal care.		
3. Use gestures. Attempt to have residents imitate the activity you want them to perform (e.g., put a fork in your mouth.) If ineffective, use hand-over-hand technique.		
4. Use eye contact and commands such as "do" and "let's." Avoid words such as "don't."		
5. Offer fluids frequently.		
6. Observe for signs of frustration and anxiety and change activity if observed. If the resident is having an episode of anxiety or agitation, gently attempt to calm the resident and refocus attention.		
7. Involve in low-stress (low-expectation) activities such as small group activities.		
8. Monitor the weights and appetite, as confused residents sometimes forget to eat.		

Self-assessment	Evaluation/ validation methods	Levels	Type of validation	Comments
❏ Experienced ❏ Need practice ❏ Never done ❏ Not applicable (based on scope of practice)	❏ Verbal ❏ Demonstration/ observation ❏ Practical exercise ❏ Interactive class	❏ Beginner ❏ Intermediate ❏ Expert	❏ Orientation ❏ Annual ❏ Other _____	

_____ _____
Employee signature   **Observer signature**

Name: _____ Date: _____

Skill: **Clean Dressing Application**

Steps	Completed	Comments
1. Explain the reason and procedure to the resident.		
2. Wash your hands and pull the curtain.		
3. Put on gloves.		
4. Remove the soiled dressing. Discard in plastic bag or according to facility policy. Avoid crossing over clean supplies with soiled items.		
5. Cleanse wound with the solution ordered. Always clean the area from the center out or from the cleanest to least clean area.		
6. Remove and discard gloves. Wash bandage scissors with soap and water if used during soiled part of procedure. Wash hands. Apply new gloves.		
7. Apply the dressing.		
8. Remove your gloves.		
9. Discard soiled items according to facility policy.		
10. Wash your hands. Wash bandage scissors, if used.		
11. Document changes in wound size, redness, pain, swelling, or drainage.		

Self-assessment	Evaluation/ validation methods	Levels	Type of validation	Comments
❏ Experienced ❏ Need practice ❏ Never done ❏ Not applicable (based on scope of practice)	❏ Verbal ❏ Demonstration/ observation ❏ Practical exercise ❏ Interactive class	❏ Beginner ❏ Intermediate ❏ Expert	❏ Orientation ❏ Annual ❏ Other _____	

Employee signature _____   **Observer signature** _____

Name: _____ Date: _____

Skill: **Sterile Dressing Application**

Steps	Completed	Comments
1. Explain the reason and procedure to the resident.		
2. Wash your hands and pull the curtain.		
3. Put on your gloves.		
4. Remove the soiled dressing. Discard in plastic bag or according to facility policy. Avoid crossing over clean supplies with soiled items.		
5. Cleanse wound with the solution ordered. Always clean the area from the center out.		
6. Change your gloves.		
7. Apply the sterile dressing.		
8. Remove your gloves.		
9. Remove the soiled dressings and discard per facility policy.		
10. Wash your hands.		
11. Monitor the wound for change in size, redness, pain, swelling, or drainage.		

Self-assessment	Evaluation/ validation methods	Levels	Type of validation	Comments
❏ Experienced ❏ Need practice ❏ Never done ❏ Not applicable (based on scope of practice)	❏ Verbal ❏ Demonstration/ observation ❏ Practical exercise ❏ Interactive class	❏ Beginner ❏ Intermediate ❏ Expert	❏ Orientation ❏ Annual ❏ Other _____	

_____
Employee signature

_____
Observer signature

Name: _____ Date: _____

Skill: **Cleansing Enema**

Steps	Completed	Comments
1. Explain the reason and procedure to the resident.		
2. Describe how to prepare solution, amount, temperature, etc.		
3. Wash your hands and pull the curtain.		
4. Position the resident on his or her left side with his or her right leg bent up slightly.		
5. Place a pad under the buttocks.		
6. Put on your gloves.		
7. Lubricate the tip of the tubing with water-soluble jelly and insert the tip into the anus 2 to 3 inches. Stop immediately if any resistance or pain is felt and report it to the charge nurse.		
8. Unclamp the container and slowly administer the solution until all the solution has been given. Encourage the resident to retain the solution for 10 to 20 minutes, if possible.		
9. Assist the resident on the bedpan or toilet to expel the enema.		
10. Discard equipment and clean the resident.		
11. Remove your gloves.		
12. Position the resident for comfort.		
13. Wash your hands.		

Self-assessment	Evaluation/ validation methods	Levels	Type of validation	Comments
❑ Experienced ❑ Need practice ❑ Never done ❑ Not applicable (based on scope of practice)	❑ Verbal ❑ Demonstration/ observation ❑ Practical exercise ❑ Interactive class	❑ Beginner ❑ Intermediate ❑ Expert	❑ Orientation ❑ Annual ❑ Other _____	

_____
Employee signature

_____
Observer signature

Name: _____ Date: _____

Skill: **Prefilled Enema**

Steps	Completed	Comments
1. Explain the reason and procedure to the resident.		
2. Wash your hands and pull the curtain.		
3. Position the resident on his or her left side with his or her right leg bent up slightly.		
4. Place a pad under the buttocks.		
5. Put on your gloves.		
6. Lubricate the tip of the squeeze bottle and insert the tip into the anus. Stop immediately if there is any pain or resistance is felt and report it to the charge nurse.		
7. Squeeze the container slowly until all the solution has been given.		
8. Encourage the resident to retain the solution for 10 to 20 minutes, if possible.		
9. Assist the resident on the bedpan or toilet to expel the enema.		
10. Discard equipment and clean the resident.		
11. Remove your gloves.		
12. Position the resident for comfort.		
13. Wash your hands.		

Self-assessment	Evaluation/ validation methods	Levels	Type of validation	Comments
❏ Experienced ❏ Need practice ❏ Never done ❏ Not applicable (based on scope of practice)	❏ Verbal ❏ Demonstration/ observation ❏ Practical exercise ❏ Interactive class	❏ Beginner ❏ Intermediate ❏ Expert	❏ Orientation ❏ Annual ❏ Other _____	

_____ _____
Employee signature   **Observer signature**

Name: _____ Date: _____

Skill: **Care of a Resident with Fragile Skin**

Steps	Completed	Comments
1. Turn and reposition with devices at least every two hours.		
2. Keep clean and dry. Lubricate if necessary.		
3. Encourage 80–100% of diet as ordered.		
4. Consider providing pressure-relieving mattress.		
5. Dietary will assess diet, vitamins, and mineral supplements.		
6. Provide lab tests as ordered.		
7. Provide O.O.B. daily to tolerance.		
8. Staff giving care should provide ROM.		
9. Monitor need for padding to side rails or wheel chairs.		
10. Monitor for discoloration, bruises, swelling, skin tears, redness, and report promptly.		
11. Pay special attention when moving the resident.		

Self-assessment	Evaluation/ validation methods	Levels	Type of validation	Comments
❑ Experienced ❑ Need practice ❑ Never done ❑ Not applicable (based on scope of practice)	❑ Verbal ❑ Demonstration/ observation ❑ Practical exercise ❑ Interactive class	❑ Beginner ❑ Intermediate ❑ Expert	❑ Orientation ❑ Annual ❑ Other _____	

Employee signature _____   **Observer signature** _____

Name: _____ Date: _____

Skill: **Gait Belt**

Steps	Completed	Comments
1. Explain the procedure to the resident.		
2. Securely apply the gait belt around the resident's waist.		
3. Walk along the side of the resident while holding the belt securely in the back with an underhand grasp.		
4. If the resident stumbles or loses balance, lean the resident erect or toward you to stabilize the resident.		

Self-assessment	Evaluation/ validation methods	Levels	Type of validation	Comments
❏ Experienced ❏ Need practice ❏ Never done ❏ Not applicable (based on scope of practice)	❏ Verbal ❏ Demonstration/ observation ❏ Practical exercise ❏ Interactive class	❏ Beginner ❏ Intermediate ❏ Expert	❏ Orientation ❏ Annual ❏ Other _____	

_____
Employee signature

_____
Observer signature

Name: _____ Date: _____

Skill: **Gastrostomy Feedings**

Steps	Completed	Comments
1. Explain the reason and procedure to the resident.		
2. Wash your hands.		
3. Elevate the head of the bed 30 to 45 degrees during and for one hour after the feeding.		
4. Check the placement of the tube.		
5. Hang the prescribed feeding.		
6. Ensure that the pump is set at the prescribed rate.		
7. Write the date and time on the feeding solution container.		
8. Wash your hands.		
9. Position the resident for comfort with his or her head elevated.		

Self-assessment	Evaluation/ validation methods	Levels	Type of validation	Comments
❏ Experienced ❏ Need practice ❏ Never done ❏ Not applicable (based on scope of practice)	❏ Verbal ❏ Demonstration/ observation ❏ Practical exercise ❏ Interactive class	❏ Beginner ❏ Intermediate ❏ Expert	❏ Orientation ❏ Annual ❏ Other _____	

_____
Employee signature

_____
Observer signature

 Competency Management in Long-Term Care

Name: _____ Date: _____

Skill: **Gastrostomy Tube Insertions**

Steps	Completed	Comments
1. Explain the reason and procedure to the resident.		
2. Wash your hands and pull the curtain.		
3. Lubricate the tip of the tube.		
4. Put on your gloves.		
5. Gently and slowly insert the tube into the resident's ostomy site.		
6. Check the placement of the tube. If the placement check is successful, inflate the balloon the pre-scribed amount.		
7. Remove your gloves.		
8. Attach the feeding solution.		
9. Position the resident for comfort with his or her head elevated.		
10. Wash your hands.		

Self-assessment	Evaluation/ validation methods	Levels	Type of validation	Comments
❏ Experienced ❏ Need practice ❏ Never done ❏ Not applicable (based on scope of practice)	❏ Verbal ❏ Demonstration/ observation ❏ Practical exercise ❏ Interactive class	❏ Beginner ❏ Intermediate ❏ Expert	❏ Orientation ❏ Annual ❏ Other _____	

_____
Employee signature

_____
Observer signature

Name: _____ Date: _____

Skill: **Checking the Placement of a Gastrostomy Feeding Tube**

Steps	Completed	Comments
1. Explain the reason and procedure to the resident.		
2. Wash your hands and pull the curtain.		
3. Slowly aspirate a small amount of feeding solution or gastric juices. If nothing returns, call your supervisor.		
4. If you aspirate feeding, continue feeding or medication insertion through the tube.		
5. Position the resident for comfort.		
6. Wash your hands.		

Self-assessment	Evaluation/ validation methods	Levels	Type of validation	Comments
❑ Experienced ❑ Need practice ❑ Never done ❑ Not applicable (based on scope of practice)	❑ Verbal ❑ Demonstration/ observation ❑ Practical exercise ❑ Interactive class	❑ Beginner ❑ Intermediate ❑ Expert	❑ Orientation ❑ Annual ❑ Other _____	

_____   _____
Employee signature   **Observer signature**

Name: _____   Date: _____

Skill: **Gastrostomy Tube Removal**

Steps	Completed	Comments
1. Explain the reason and procedure to the resident.		
2. Wash your hands and pull the curtain.		
3. Assist the resident into the supine position.		
4. Occlude the tube.		
5. Put on your gloves.		
6. Aspirate the sterile water from the balloon.		
7. Gently and slowly pull the tube out.		
8. Dispose of the tube per facility policy.		
9. Remove your gloves.		
10. Position the resident comfortably.		
11. Wash your hands.		

Self-assessment	Evaluation/ validation methods	Levels	Type of validation	Comments
❏ Experienced ❏ Need practice ❏ Never done ❏ Not applicable (based on scope of practice)	❏ Verbal ❏ Demonstration/ observation ❏ Practical exercise ❏ Interactive class	❏ Beginner ❏ Intermediate ❏ Expert	❏ Orientation ❏ Annual ❏ Other _____	

_____
Employee signature

_____
Observer signature

Name: _____ Date: _____

Skill: **Hearing Aid Care**

Steps	Completed	Comments
1. Explain the reason and procedure to the resident.		
2. Wash your hands.		
To insert the hearing aid: • Turn the hearing aid off • Rotate the ear mold gently and place in the ear canal • Turn the aid on and set the hearing aid's volume up to where the resident feels comfortable		
To remove the hearing aid: • Turn the hearing aid off. • Remove the mold gently from the ear. • Ensure that it isn't soiled. Wipe with a damp cloth if it is soiled. • Return the aid to its case.		
3. Wash your hands.		
4. Change the batteries when the aid is not effective.		
5. Ensure that the aid is removed prior to a shower or shampoo, using an electric razor or hair dryer.		

Self-assessment	Evaluation/ validation methods	Levels	Type of validation	Comments
❏ Experienced ❏ Need practice ❏ Never done ❏ Not applicable (based on scope of practice)	❏ Verbal ❏ Demonstration/ observation ❏ Practical exercise ❏ Interactive class	❏ Beginner ❏ Intermediate ❏ Expert	❏ Orientation ❏ Annual ❏ Other _____	

_____   _____
Employee signature   **Observer signature**

Name:	Date:

Skill: **Heimlich Maneuver**

Steps	Completed	Comments
1. Stand behind the resident.		
2. Wrap your arms around the resident's waist.		
3. Bend the resident slightly forward.		
4. Place your hands below the rib cage and sternum with one hand in a fist and the other hand holding it.		
5. Briskly pull your hands inward and upward.		
6. Repeat the action several times until the article obstructing the airway is discharged.		
7. Continue until obstruction is freed or resident loses consciousness. (Follow with unconscious procedure.)		

Self-assessment	Evaluation/ validation methods	Levels	Type of validation	Comments
❑ Experienced ❑ Need practice ❑ Never done ❑ Not applicable (based on scope of practice)	❑ Verbal ❑ Demonstration/ observation ❑ Practical exercise ❑ Interactive class	❑ Beginner ❑ Intermediate ❑ Expert	❑ Orientation ❑ Annual ❑ Other _____	

_____
Employee signature

_____
Observer signature

Name: _____ Date: _____

Skill: **Mechanical Lift**

Steps	Completed	Comments
1. Explain the reason and procedure to the resident.		
2. Wash your hands and pull the curtain.		
3. Place the seat under the resident with the wider portion under the resident's thighs and buttocks.		
4. Raise the head of the bed.		
5. Place the base of the lift under the bed.		
6. Attach the seat to the lift.		
7. Turn the handle to lift the resident.		
8. When the lift is high enough over the bed to move the resident, then roll the lift away from the bed and over the chair.		
9. Slowly lower the resident into the chair.		
10. Unhook the seat from the lift and leave the seat under the resident. Ensure that the seat isn't wrinkled up under the resident.		
11. Reverse the above to return the resident to bed.		

Self-assessment	Evaluation/ validation methods	Levels	Type of validation	Comments
❏ Experienced ❏ Need practice ❏ Never done ❏ Not applicable (based on scope of practice)	❏ Verbal ❏ Demonstration/ observation ❏ Practical exercise ❏ Interactive class	❏ Beginner ❏ Intermediate ❏ Expert	❏ Orientation ❏ Annual ❏ Other _____	

_____
Employee signature

_____
Observer signature

Name: _____ Date: _____

Skill: **Prefilled Oxygen Humidifiers**

Steps	Completed	Comments
1. Explain the reason and procedure to the resident.		
2. Wash your hands.		
3. Remove sterile unit from its wrapping.		
4. Remove the caps from the unit.		
5. Attach the humidifier to the flowmeter or the concentrator.		
6. Attach the humidifier to the tubing.		
7. Adjust the oxygen flow rate.		
8. Ensure that the oxygen is flowing out of the tubing.		
9. Position cannula or mask on the resident.		
10. Monitor to ensure that it is functioning properly.		
11. Date, time, and initial the unit. Change every _____ days.		

Self-assessment	Evaluation/ validation methods	Levels	Type of validation	Comments
❑ Experienced ❑ Need practice ❑ Never done ❑ Not applicable (based on scope of practice)	❑ Verbal ❑ Demonstration/ observation ❑ Practical exercise ❑ Interactive class	❑ Beginner ❑ Intermediate ❑ Expert	❑ Orientation ❑ Annual ❑ Other _____	

_____   _____
Employee signature   **Observer signature**

Name: _____ Date: _____

Skill: **Intramuscular Injections**

Steps	Completed	Comments
1. Check the medication sheet for the last site used.		
2. Wipe the top of the medication vial with an alcohol wipe. Fill the syringe with the correct amount of ordered medication.		
3. Replace the needle protector.		
4. Identify the resident.		
5. Explain the reason and procedure to the resident.		
6. Wash your hands and pull the curtain.		
7. Cleanse the injection site with an alcohol swab.		
8. Insert the needle quickly at right angles.		
9. Aspirate slightly before injecting. If there is any blood, withdraw the needle and prepare another injection.		
10. Inject the solution slowly.		
11. Place an alcohol sponge over the site and withdraw the needle.		
12. Massage the site slightly. Monitor site for blood, pain, or irritation.		
13. Position the resident for comfort.		
14. Dispose of the needle in the sharps container. Do not recap the needle.		
15. Wash your hands.		
16. Record in the resident's record.		

Self-assessment	Evaluation/ validation methods	Levels	Type of validation	Comments
❏ Experienced ❏ Need practice ❏ Never done ❏ Not applicable (based on scope of practice)	❏ Verbal ❏ Demonstration/ observation ❏ Practical exercise ❏ Interactive class	❏ Beginner ❏ Intermediate ❏ Expert	❏ Orientation ❏ Annual ❏ Other _____	

Employee signature _____

Observer signature _____

Name: _____ Date: _____

Skill: **Subcutaneous Injections**

Steps	Completed	Comments
1. Check the medication sheet for the last site used.		
2. Wipe of the top of the medication vial with an alcohol wipe. Fill the syringe with the correct amount of ordered medication.		
3. Replace the needle protector.		
4. Identify the resident.		
5. Explain the reason and procedure to the resident.		
6. Pull the curtain.		
7. Cleanse the injection site with an alcohol swab.		
8. Hold a section of the skin with your thumb and index finger and raise it to elevate the subcutaneous tissue. Insert the needle quickly at a 45-degree angle.		
9. Aspirate slightly before injecting. If there is any blood, withdraw the needle and prepare another injection.		
10. Inject the solution slowly.		
11. Place an alcohol sponge over the site and withdraw the needle.		
12. Massage the site slightly. Monitor site for blood, pain, or irritation.		
13. Position the resident for comfort.		
14. Dispose of the needle in the sharps container. Do not recap the needle.		
15. Wash your hands.		
16. Record in the resident's record.		

Self-assessment	Evaluation/ validation methods	Levels	Type of validation	Comments
❏ Experienced ❏ Need practice ❏ Never done ❏ Not applicable (based on scope of practice)	❏ Verbal ❏ Demonstration/ observation ❏ Practical exercise ❏ Interactive class	❏ Beginner ❏ Intermediate ❏ Expert	❏ Orientation ❏ Annual ❏ Other _____	

Employee signature _____

Observer signature _____

Name: _____ Date: _____

Skill: **Care of the Resident with Insomnia**

Steps	Completed	Comments
1. Ensure that there is a quiet environment.		
2. Encourage the resident to stay up during day for sleep at night.		
3. Monitor for and identify causes for insomnia: medications, caffeine, over stimulation, depression, anxiety. If a cause is identified, develop a plan of care to eliminate it or minimize its effect on the resident's sleep pattern.		
4. Medication as ordered and needed. Monitor for drowsiness the morning following medication administration.		
5. Encourage activity attendance during the day.		
6. If the resident is awake and agitated during the night, monitor for getting out of bed.		

Self-assessment	Evaluation/ validation methods	Levels	Type of validation	Comments
❏ Experienced ❏ Need practice ❏ Never done ❏ Not applicable (based on scope of practice)	❏ Verbal ❏ Demonstration/ observation ❏ Practical exercise ❏ Interactive class	❏ Beginner ❏ Intermediate ❏ Expert	❏ Orientation ❏ Annual ❏ Other _____	

_____   _____
Employee signature   **Observer signature**

   Competency Management in Long-Term Care

Name: _____ Date: _____

Skill: **Lab Result Reporting**

Steps	Completed	Comments
1. When an abnormal lab or X-ray result is reported by phone, the charge nurse will call the physician's office and report the results. The nurse will chart this notification in the nurses' notes.		
2. When an abnormal lab or X-ray result is reported by fax, the charge nurse will call the physician's office and report the results. The nurse may then fax the report to the physician.		
3. These actions will be charted on the laboratory or X-ray report, if available. (With a phone report, no written report is available.)		

Self-assessment	Evaluation/ validation methods	Levels	Type of validation	Comments
❑ Experienced ❑ Need practice ❑ Never done ❑ Not applicable (based on scope of practice)	❑ Verbal ❑ Demonstration/ observation ❑ Practical exercise ❑ Interactive class	❑ Beginner ❑ Intermediate ❑ Expert	❑ Orientation ❑ Annual ❑ Other _____	

_____   _____
Employee signature   **Observer signature**

Name: _____ Date: _____

Skill: **Linen Handling**

Steps	Completed	Comments
1. Take only linen needed for a specific resident into the room and place it on the resident's clean over-bed table.		
2. Remove the soiled linen from the bed.		
3. Deposit soiled linen directly into the covered linen receptacle or plastic bag. Never place soiled linen on the floor, over bed table, bedside stand, or chair. Keep the soiled linen container covered.		
4. Wash your hands prior to handling clean linen.		
5. Personal laundry should be placed in the designated waterproof container. Never hang soiled clothing in the resident's closet.		
6. Remove soiled linen containers from the hallway during meal times.		
7. Transport soiled linen containers to the laundry when they are full.		

Self-assessment	Evaluation/ validation methods	Levels	Type of validation	Comments
❏ Experienced ❏ Need practice ❏ Never done ❏ Not applicable (based on scope of practice)	❏ Verbal ❏ Demonstration/ observation ❏ Practical exercise ❏ Interactive class	❏ Beginner ❏ Intermediate ❏ Expert	❏ Orientation ❏ Annual ❏ Other _____	

_____   _____

Employee signature   **Observer signature**

Name: _____ Date: _____

Skill: **Medication Administration**

Steps	Completed	Comments
1. Check the medication administration sheet.		
2. Pour the medication without touching the inside of the container. Shake all liquids well. If the resident is unable to swallow, crush the medications and put in applesauce unless contraindicated. (A physicians' order is needed to routinely administer crushed medications. Use a liquid preparation instead, if available. If the medication is given through a tube, order the medication in liquid form, if possible. If not, crush and put in enough water to enable administration through the tube. Inject 30 to 50 ml water into tube before and after each medication is administered.		
3. Identify the resident.		
4. If vital sign or blood sugar monitoring are ordered, perform prior to giving medications.		
5. Administer the medication. Ensure that the resident has enough fluids to swallow his or her medication. Never leave medication at the bedside.		
6. Chart the medication given.		
7. Use a sanitizing solution to cleanse hands between residents. Wash your hands, if soiled, and after ear or eye drops are administered.		
8. Monitor for side effects for all medications given.		
9. Medications are to be given within one hour prior to or after time ordered.		
10. Medication carts are to be locked when out of the sight of a licensed nurse.		
11. Medication carts are to be kept clean at all times.		

Self-assessment	Evaluation/ validation methods	Levels	Type of validation	Comments
❏ Experienced ❏ Need practice ❏ Never done ❏ Not applicable (based on scope of practice)	❏ Verbal ❏ Demonstration/ observation ❏ Practical exercise ❏ Interactive class	❏ Beginner ❏ Intermediate ❏ Expert	❏ Orientation ❏ Annual ❏ Other _____	

_____   _____
Employee signature   **Observer signature**

Name: _____ Date: _____

Skill: **Medication Errors**

Steps	Completed	Comments
1. Notify the attending physician and resident or responsible party.		
2. Follow any physician orders.		
3. Document on a medication error form or incident report, according to facility policy.		
4. Monitor the resident closely for 24 hours and report any changes to the attending physician.		

Self-assessment	Evaluation/ validation methods	Levels	Type of validation	Comments
❏ Experienced ❏ Need practice ❏ Never done ❏ Not applicable (based on scope of practice)	❏ Verbal ❏ Demonstration/ observation ❏ Practical exercise ❏ Interactive class	❏ Beginner ❏ Intermediate ❏ Expert	❏ Orientation ❏ Annual ❏ Other _____	

_____   _____
Employee signature   **Observer signature**

Name: _____ Date: _____

Skill: **Missing Resident**

Steps	Completed	Comments
1. Notify the charge nurse.		
2. Notify the supervisor or administrator on duty.		
3. A search of all the rooms in the facility (including utility rooms and service areas) will be done if a resident is thought to be missing. Check under beds, closets, bathroom, and shower and tub rooms. Assign two persons to check each hallway, one on each side. The location of each resident will be verified.		
4. Assign two personnel to check the area immediately outside the facility. Personnel should go around the facility in opposite directions. When they meet, they should return inside for reassignment.		
5. Assign two personnel to check the kitchen, basement, lobby, activity room, chapel, elevator, stairwells, and offices.		
6. Assign available staff to begin a search of the neighborhood. (Some staff members should always remain in the building with residents.)		
7. If the resident has not been found within 15 minutes, or after a search of the facility and immediately outside the building, the person in charge shall carry out these steps: • Notify the police or local law enforcement agency. • Notify the family or responsible party. Explain what is being done to find the resident. • Notify other regulatory agencies, as required by law.		
8. When law enforcement arrives, give them: • Resident's name, nickname, gender, age, height, weight, race, hair and eye color, mental condition, and language spoken • Description of clothing • Picture of the resident • Former address, or possible location, if known • Other information that will assist in determining the resident's whereabouts • The authorities may assume command and direction of the search from this point		

9. Upon return of the resident to the facility, the charge nurse or director of nursing will:
 	
• Completely assess the resident for injuries and contact the attending physician and report findings and condition of the resident.
 	
• Notify all previously contacted persons and organizations of the return of the resident.
 	
• Complete an incident report detailing the incident in its entirety.
 	
• Document the incident in the resident's chart. Documentation should be objective and concise and reflect the actual facts as they relate to the incident, including:
    – Times
    – Persons contacted
    – Missing person's physical, mental and emotional status prior to event
    – Details such as last seen, staff actions, status of how, when, and where found, condition
    – Assessment of injuries, condition of resident upon return to the facility, clothing, temperature outside, areas of skin exposed, etc.
    – Physician notification
    – Physician's orders
    – Treatment given, if any
    – Other pertinent information
 	
• Review and revise/update the care plan to reflect the incident and modify approaches to prevent recurrence. Consider whether a significant change MDS should be done.		

     Competency Management in Long-Term Care

10. Quality Assurance. A complete and thorough root-cause analysis of the elopement should be done to prevent recurrence; to ensure policies, procedures, and systems are effective; and to protect other residents. Questions that need to be asked may include: • Were the alarm systems working properly? • Were all internal and external doors visually checked? • Were there any deficient practices or system failures? • What is being done to prevent recurrence? All root-cause analysis information should be summarized and discussed at the next quality assurance meeting. Records should be kept of all incidents so that trends and risks can be identified and reduced. Other QA functions include: • Randomly test door and personal alarm systems • Stage quarterly mock drills to test compliance of the plan • Review policies and procedures and make recommendations for updates.		

Self-assessment	Evaluation/ validation methods	Levels	Type of validation	Comments
❏ Experienced ❏ Need practice ❏ Never done ❏ Not applicable (based on scope of practice)	❏ Verbal ❏ Demonstration/ observation ❏ Practical exercise ❏ Interactive class	❏ Beginner ❏ Intermediate ❏ Expert	❏ Orientation ❏ Annual ❏ Other _____	

Employee signature

Observer signature

| Name: | | Date: | |

Skill: **Postmortem Care: Preparing the Body**

Steps	Completed	Comments
1. Ensure that the deceased resident is in an empty room.		
2. Wash your hands and pull the curtain. Apply the principles of standard precautions. The body can be infectious after death.		
3. Gently pull the eyelashes down to close the resident's eyes.		
4. Remove all tubes.		
5. Insert the resident's dentures, if available, or send to the funeral home with the body.		
6. Ensure that the resident's identification bracelet is on and readable.		
7. Bathe the resident.		
8. Replace all dressings with clean dressings.		
9. Place a clean pad under the resident's buttocks.		
10. Wash your hands.		
11. Assist the mortuary when they arrive. Have the mortuary sign a receipt for the body.		
12. Follow facility policy for disposition of medications and personal belongings. Remove medications from the active supply and store in the designated area. Bag the resident's belongings for pickup by the responsible party.		

Self-assessment	Evaluation/ validation methods	Levels	Type of validation	Comments
❑ Experienced ❑ Need practice ❑ Never done ❑ Not applicable (based on scope of practice)	❑ Verbal ❑ Demonstration/ observation ❑ Practical exercise ❑ Interactive class	❑ Beginner ❑ Intermediate ❑ Expert	❑ Orientation ❑ Annual ❑ Other _____	

Employee signature

Observer signature

| Name: _____ | Date: _____ |

Skill: **Postmortem Care: Licensed Nurse**

Steps	Completed	Comments
1. Ensure that the deceased resident is in an empty room.		
2. Notify the attending physician of the lack of vital signs. Ask for a discharge body to mortuary order. Ask whether the physician will notify the family.		
3. Notify the responsible party, if requested by the physician. Notify the coroner or justice of the peace, if required in your locale.		
4. Pronounce the resident and document your assessment, if permitted by state law.		
5. Notify the mortuary.		
6. Have the mortuary sign the discharge receipt for the resident.		
7. Chart the time and specific person notified in steps 2, 3, and 5.		
8. Chart the condition of the body when discharged: pressure ulcers, bruises, rings. Ensure that jewelry is mentioned by color, not assumed metal type.		

Self-assessment	Evaluation/ validation methods	Levels	Type of validation	Comments
❏ Experienced ❏ Need practice ❏ Never done ❏ Not applicable (based on scope of practice)	❏ Verbal ❏ Demonstration/ observation ❏ Practical exercise ❏ Interactive class	❏ Beginner ❏ Intermediate ❏ Expert	❏ Orientation ❏ Annual ❏ Other _____	

_____
Employee signature

_____
Observer signature

Name: _____ Date: _____

Skill: **Nasogastric Tube Feedings**

Steps	Completed	Comments
1. Explain the reason and procedure to the resident.		
2. Wash your hands.		
3. Assure that the resident's head is elevated.		
4. Check the placement of the tube.		
5. Hang the prescribed feeding.		
6. Assure that the pump is set at the prescribed rate.		
7. Write the date and time on the feeding solution container.		
8. Wash your hands.		
9. Position the resident for comfort with his or her head elevated.		
10. Monitor the resident frequently to ensure that he or she is repositioned with his or her head elevated to prevent aspiration.		

Self-assessment	Evaluation/ validation methods	Levels	Type of validation	Comments
❏ Experienced ❏ Need practice ❏ Never done ❏ Not applicable (based on scope of practice)	❏ Verbal ❏ Demonstration/ observation ❏ Practical exercise ❏ Interactive class	❏ Beginner ❏ Intermediate ❏ Expert	❏ Orientation ❏ Annual ❏ Other _____	

_____
Employee signature

_____
Observer signature

Name: _____   Date: _____

Skill: **Nasogastric Tube Insertion**

Steps	Completed	Comments
1. Explain the reason and procedure to the resident.		
2. Wash your hands and pull the curtain.		
3. Assist the resident into a semi-Fowler's position.		
4. Place a pad under the resident's chin.		
5. Put on your gloves.		
6. Lubricate the tip of the tube.		
7. Gently and slowly insert the tube into the resident's nostril.		
8. Instruct the resident to swallow repeatedly.		
9. Stop and remove the tube immediately if you encounter resistance, the resident starts coughing, you can hear air escape the tube, or the resident's color changes and call a supervisor.		
10. Check the placement of the tube.		
11. Secure the tube to the nose with tape. Ensure that the tube is not in the resident's range of sight.		
12. Remove your gloves.		
13. Position the resident for comfort with his or her head elevated.		
14. Wash your hands.		

Self-assessment	Evaluation/ validation methods	Levels	Type of validation	Comments
❏ Experienced ❏ Need practice ❏ Never done ❏ Not applicable (based on scope of practice)	❏ Verbal ❏ Demonstration/ observation ❏ Practical exercise ❏ Interactive class	❏ Beginner ❏ Intermediate ❏ Expert	❏ Orientation ❏ Annual ❏ Other _____	

_____
Employee signature

_____
Observer signature

Name: _____ Date: _____

Skill: **Checking the Placement of a Nasogastric Feeding Tube**

Steps	Completed	Comments
1. Explain the reason and procedure to the resident.		
2. Wash your hands and pull the curtain.		
3. Place the stethoscope over the resident's stomach.		
4. Put on your gloves.		
5. Inject a small amount of air through the tube. You should hear air sounds in the tube. If you hear nothing, don't put anything in the tube and call a supervisor.		
6. Slowly aspirate a small amount of feeding solution or gastric juices. If nothing returns, call your supervisor.		
7. If you hear air sounds and aspirate feeding, continue feeding or medication insertion through the tube.		
8. Remove your gloves.		
9. Position the resident for comfort.		
10. Wash your hands.		

Self-assessment	Evaluation/ validation methods	Levels	Type of validation	Comments
❑ Experienced ❑ Need practice ❑ Never done ❑ Not applicable (based on scope of practice)	❑ Verbal ❑ Demonstration/ observation ❑ Practical exercise ❑ Interactive class	❑ Beginner ❑ Intermediate ❑ Expert	❑ Orientation ❑ Annual ❑ Other _____	

_____
Employee signature

_____
Observer signature

Name: _____   Date: _____

Skill: **Nasogastric Tube Removal**

Steps	Completed	Comments
1. Explain the reason and procedure to the resident.		
2. Wash your hands and pull the curtain.		
3. Assist the resident into a semi-Fowler's position.		
4. Place a pad or towel under the resident's chin.		
5. Put on your gloves.		
6. Occlude the tube.		
7. Gently and slowly pull the tube out.		
8. Dispose of the tube per facility policy.		
9. Remove your gloves.		
10. Position the resident comfortably.		
11. Wash your hands.		

Self-assessment	Evaluation/ validation methods	Levels	Type of validation	Comments
❏ Experienced ❏ Need practice ❏ Never done ❏ Not applicable (based on scope of practice)	❏ Verbal ❏ Demonstration/ observation ❏ Practical exercise ❏ Interactive class	❏ Beginner ❏ Intermediate ❏ Expert	❏ Orientation ❏ Annual ❏ Other _____	

_____
Employee signature

_____
Observer signature

Name: _____ Date: _____

Skill: **Oral Hygiene**

Steps	Completed	Comments
1. Explain the reason and procedure to the resident.		
2. Wash your hands.		
3. Wet and place a small amount of toothpaste on the toothbrush.		
4. Place an emesis basin under the resident's chin.		
5. Assist the resident in brushing the teeth.		
6. Assist the resident in rinsing the mouth with water.		
7. Empty and rinse the emesis basin.		
8. Wash your hands.		

Self-assessment	Evaluation/ validation methods	Levels	Type of validation	Comments
❏ Experienced ❏ Need practice ❏ Never done ❏ Not applicable (based on scope of practice)	❏ Verbal ❏ Demonstration/ observation ❏ Practical exercise ❏ Interactive class	❏ Beginner ❏ Intermediate ❏ Expert	❏ Orientation ❏ Annual ❏ Other _____	

_____
Employee signature

_____
Observer signature

  Competency Management in Long-Term Care

Name: _____ Date: _____

Skill: **Oral Hygiene for Unconscious Residents**

Steps	Completed	Comments
1. Explain the reason and procedure to the resident.		
2. Wash your hands.		
3. Place the resident on one side with a towel underneath the cheek.		
4. Moisten a sponge applicator (Toothette®). Squeeze to remove excess water.		
5. Gently wipe inside of the resident's mouth.		
6. Rinse the resident's mouth with a damp sponge applicator.		
7. Lubricate the resident's mouth and lips with lip balm or petroleum jelly.		
8. Position the resident.		
9. Wash your hands.		

Self-assessment	Evaluation/ validation methods	Levels	Type of validation	Comments
❑ Experienced ❑ Need practice ❑ Never done ❑ Not applicable (based on scope of practice)	❑ Verbal ❑ Demonstration/ observation ❑ Practical exercise ❑ Interactive class	❑ Beginner ❑ Intermediate ❑ Expert	❑ Orientation ❑ Annual ❑ Other _____	

_____
Employee signature

_____
Observer signature

Name: _____ Date: _____

Skill: **Oxygen Administration**

Steps	Completed	Comments
1. Explain the reason and procedure to the resident.		
2. Wash your hands.		
3. Date the humidifier bottle.		
4. Turn oxygen on the prescribed amount. Test that oxygen is coming out of mask or cannula.		
5. Place the cannula or mask on the resident.		
6. Instruct the resident to breathe normally.		
7. Wash your hands.		
8. Place the "Oxygen in Use" sign on the resident's doorway and above the head of the bed, or according to facility policy.		
9. Ensure that humidifiers are changed every __ days or when the fluid falls below the minimum fill line.		

Self-assessment	Evaluation/ validation methods	Levels	Type of validation	Comments
❑ Experienced ❑ Need practice ❑ Never done ❑ Not applicable (based on scope of practice)	❑ Verbal ❑ Demonstration/ observation ❑ Practical exercise ❑ Interactive class	❑ Beginner ❑ Intermediate ❑ Expert	❑ Orientation ❑ Annual ❑ Other _____	

_____
Employee signature

_____
Observer signature

Name: _____ Date: _____

Skill: **Pacemaker Checks**

Steps	Completed	Comments
1. Explain the reason and procedure to the resident.		
2. Assist the resident to the telephone area on the scheduled date.		
3. Attach the pacemaker analysis machine to the phone according to manufacturer's directions.		
4. Dial the phone number. Run the test.		
5. Record the results in the chart. Notify the physician if there is a problem.		

Self-assessment	Evaluation/ validation methods	Levels	Type of validation	Comments
❏ Experienced ❏ Need practice ❏ Never done ❏ Not applicable (based on scope of practice)	❏ Verbal ❏ Demonstration/ observation ❏ Practical exercise ❏ Interactive class	❏ Beginner ❏ Intermediate ❏ Expert	❏ Orientation ❏ Annual ❏ Other _____	

Employee signature _____ **Observer signature** _____

Name: _____ Date: _____

Skill: **Psychotherapeutic Medication Use**

Steps	Completed	Comments
1. Explain the reason and possible side effects to the resident or his or her surrogate decision-maker. See consents.		
2. Give medications as ordered.		
3. Monitor for and document side effects. If present, notify the physician promptly.		
4. Monitor for and document effectiveness of the medication. If ineffective, notify the physician.		
5. Ensure that the lowest therapeutic doses are given.		

Self-assessment	Evaluation/ validation methods	Levels	Type of validation	Comments
❑ Experienced ❑ Need practice ❑ Never done ❑ Not applicable (based on scope of practice)	❑ Verbal ❑ Demonstration/ observation ❑ Practical exercise ❑ Interactive class	❑ Beginner ❑ Intermediate ❑ Expert	❑ Orientation ❑ Annual ❑ Other _____	

_____   _____
Employee signature   **Observer signature**

Name: _____ Date: _____

Skill: **Positioning**

Steps	Completed	Comments
In a bed		
1. Explain the reason and procedure to the resident.		
2. Wash your hands and pull the curtain.		
3. Change the position from the back, left side, and right side every two hours unless contraindicated.		
4. Use pillows to maintain position and prevent skin from touching skin.		
5. Use positioning devices as indicated.		
6. Report any red areas to the charge nurse promptly.		
7. Wash your hands.		
In a chair		
1. Explain the procedure.		
2. Reposition every two hours or more often, according to plan of care.		
3. Move the resident and change the points of pressure.		
4. Wash your hands.		

Self-assessment	Evaluation/ validation methods	Levels	Type of validation	Comments
❑ Experienced ❑ Need practice ❑ Never done ❑ Not applicable (based on scope of practice)	❑ Verbal ❑ Demonstration/ observation ❑ Practical exercise ❑ Interactive class	❑ Beginner ❑ Intermediate ❑ Expert	❑ Orientation ❑ Annual ❑ Other _____	

_____   _____
Employee signature   **Observer signature**

Name: _____ Date: _____

Skill: **Taking a Pulse**

Steps	Completed	Comments
Radial Pulse		
1. Explain the reason and procedure to the resident.		
2. Wash your hands.		
3. Gently press two fingers over the radial artery on the resident's wrist.		
4. Count the number of beats for 30 seconds and multiply by two. If the pulse is irregular, count for 60 seconds.		
5. Record the results.		
Apical Pulse		
1. Explain the reason and procedure to the resident.		
2. Wash your hands.		
3. Locate the resident's pulse with your stethoscope on the left side of the chest.		
4. Count the number of beats for one minute.		
5. Record the results.		

Self-assessment	Evaluation/ validation methods	Levels	Type of validation	Comments
❑ Experienced ❑ Need practice ❑ Never done ❑ Not applicable (based on scope of practice)	❑ Verbal ❑ Demonstration/ observation ❑ Practical exercise ❑ Interactive class	❑ Beginner ❑ Intermediate ❑ Expert	❑ Orientation ❑ Annual ❑ Other _____	

_____   _____

Employee signature   **Observer signature**

Name: _____ Date: _____

Skill: **Care of the Resident Receiving Radiation Treatments**

Steps	Completed	Comments
1. Encourage rest after radiation.		
2. Lab and medications as ordered with abnormals reported promptly.		
3. Notify physician if nausea or vomiting occurs.		
4. Monitor skin. Do not use soap on irradiated area or wash off radiation markings.		
5. Staff to monitor the resident, medications, diet, environment, and labs for possible complications.		
6. Encourage fluids.		
7. Medication if ordered. Report to the physician if ineffective.		
8. Visit with the resident when sick to help relieve anxiety due to treatment or side effects.		
9. Monitor diet for tolerance.		
10. Treatments as ordered.		

Self-assessment	Evaluation/ validation methods	Levels	Type of validation	Comments
❏ Experienced ❏ Need practice ❏ Never done ❏ Not applicable (based on scope of practice)	❏ Verbal ❏ Demonstration/ observation ❏ Practical exercise ❏ Interactive class	❏ Beginner ❏ Intermediate ❏ Expert	❏ Orientation ❏ Annual ❏ Other _____	

_____   _____
Employee signature   **Observer signature**

Name: _____ Date: _____

Skill: **Care of the Resident with Renal Disease**

Steps	Completed	Comments
1. Monitor the feet and hands for edema, blood pressure daily, and weight daily, weekly, or as ordered.		
2. Encourage the resident to be out of bed daily and exercise.		
3. Provide diet and medications as ordered.		
4. Notify the physician if edema, chest pain, elevated B/P or shortness of breath occur.		
5. Lab and X-ray as ordered.		
6. Good personal hygiene. Notify the physician if the resident complains of itching.		
7. Monitor I&O.		

Self-assessment	Evaluation/ validation methods	Levels	Type of validation	Comments
❏ Experienced ❏ Need practice ❏ Never done ❏ Not applicable (based on scope of practice)	❏ Verbal ❏ Demonstration/ observation ❏ Practical exercise ❏ Interactive class	❏ Beginner ❏ Intermediate ❏ Expert	❏ Orientation ❏ Annual ❏ Other _____	

_____   _____
Employee signature   **Observer signature**

          Competency Management in Long-Term Care

| Name: _____ | Date: _____ |

Skill: Range of Motion Exercises

Steps	Completed	Comments
1. Explain the reason and procedure to the resident. Position the resident in the supine position.		
2. Encourage and assist the resident in gently rotating his or her head forward, side to side, and backward.		
3. Encourage and assist the resident in gently rotating his or her arms up, down, and sideways.		
4. Encourage and assist the resident in gently bending his or her elbows back and straight out.		
5. Encourage and assist the resident in gently moving fingers from a ball to straight out. (Add scissors motion for each finger, and touch each finger to thumb.)		
6. Encourage and assist the resident in gently rotating his or her wrists up, down, around, and sideways.		
7. Encourage and assist the resident in gently rotating his or her legs up, down, and sideways. Roll the femur gently from side to side while resting on the bed.		
8. Encourage and assist the resident in alternating between gently bending his or her knees upward and straightening them out.		
9. Encourage and assist the resident in gently rotating his or her ankles up, down, sideways, and in a circle.		
10. Encourage and assist the resident in gently rotating his or her toes up and down and sideways. Spread each toe apart in a scissors motion. Bend toes down with the palm of your hand. Never move a joint beyond its limitations or as far as it will comfortably go. Consult the nurse for special instructions before exercising joints that are contracted and those which have been fractured in the past 180 days.		
11. Stop the exercises if the resident feels pain or gets dizzy.		

Self-assessment	Evaluation/ validation methods	Levels	Type of validation	Comments
❏ Experienced ❏ Need practice ❏ Never done ❏ Not applicable (based on scope of practice)	❏ Verbal ❏ Demonstration/ observation ❏ Practical exercise ❏ Interactive class	❏ Beginner ❏ Intermediate ❏ Expert	❏ Orientation ❏ Annual ❏ Other _____	

_____
Employee signature

_____
Observer signature

Name: _____ Date: _____

Skill: **Respirations**

Steps	Completed	Comments
1. While you are taking the resident's pulse, count the number of times the resident's chest rises and falls for 30 seconds. Do not tell the resident you are counting the respiratory rate.		
2. Multiply the number by two.		
3. Record the results.		

Self-assessment	Evaluation/ validation methods	Levels	Type of validation	Comments
❑ Experienced ❑ Need practice ❑ Never done ❑ Not applicable (based on scope of practice)	❑ Verbal ❑ Demonstration/ observation ❑ Practical exercise ❑ Interactive class	❑ Beginner ❑ Intermediate ❑ Expert	❑ Orientation ❑ Annual ❑ Other _____	

_____
Employee signature

_____
Observer signature

Name: _____ Date: _____

Skill: **Care of the Resident with Respiratory Disease**

Steps	Completed	Comments
1. Monitor the resident for episodes of shortness of breath and implement interventions as ordered.		
2. Monitor the feet and hands for warmth, color, or edema.		
3. Notify the physician if edema or shortness of breath occurs.		
4. Encourage the resident to be out of bed daily and exercise.		
5. Give the medications as ordered.		
6. Provide lab and X-ray as ordered.		
7. Monitor for anxiety and be present to render support to prevent anxiety if an episode of shortness of breath occurs.		
8. Encourage the resident to attend activities that do not depend on major physical stamina or exertion, such as music, games, and parties.		
9. Administer oxygen as ordered, if needed.		

Self-assessment	Evaluation/ validation methods	Levels	Type of validation	Comments
❏ Experienced ❏ Need practice ❏ Never done ❏ Not applicable (based on scope of practice)	❏ Verbal ❏ Demonstration/ observation ❏ Practical exercise ❏ Interactive class	❏ Beginner ❏ Intermediate ❏ Expert	❏ Orientation ❏ Annual ❏ Other _____	

Employee signature _____ **Observer signature** _____

Name: _____ Date: _____

Skill: **Restraints**

Steps	Completed	Comments
1. An interdisciplinary team shall assess each restrained resident for the least restrictive restraint possible. Restraints are applied only upon proper physicians' order stating type of restraint, time restraint is to be applied, reason for restraint, and release of restraint.		
2. Make sure the resident is in a comfortable position, has call signal, water, and needed personal items available before leaving the room. Visually check the resident's well-being every 15 to 30 minutes.		
3. Any restrained resident shall have the restraint released at least every two hours to prevent decreased functioning. Provide exercise, ambulation, and toileting when the restraint is released. Document application and restraint release.		
4. Restraints shall be reassessed at least quarterly by reviewing the care plan entry for the restraint.		

Self-assessment	Evaluation/ validation methods	Levels	Type of validation	Comments
❏ Experienced ❏ Need practice ❏ Never done ❏ Not applicable (based on scope of practice)	❏ Verbal ❏ Demonstration/ observation ❏ Practical exercise ❏ Interactive class	❏ Beginner ❏ Intermediate ❏ Expert	❏ Orientation ❏ Annual ❏ Other _____	

_____
Employee signature

_____
Observer signature

Name: _____   Date: _____

Skill: **Seizure Precautions**

Steps	Completed	Comments
1. If a resident is having a seizure, stay with him or her and call for help.		
2. If the resident is in bed, remove the pillow and raise the side rails. If he or she is not in a bed, lower him or her to the floor, protecting the head.		
3. If possible, turn the resident on his or her side to allow any secretions to drain.		
4. Loosen tight and restrictive clothing.		
5. Do not place any object into the resident's mouth.		
6. Check the resident's vital signs as needed.		
7. When the seizure stops, orient the resident and explain to him or her what happened.		
8. Report all seizures to the physician.		

Self-assessment	Evaluation/ validation methods	Levels	Type of validation	Comments
❑ Experienced ❑ Need practice ❑ Never done ❑ Not applicable (based on scope of practice)	❑ Verbal ❑ Demonstration/ observation ❑ Practical exercise ❑ Interactive class	❑ Beginner ❑ Intermediate ❑ Expert	❑ Orientation ❑ Annual ❑ Other _____	

_____   _____
Employee signature   **Observer signature**

Name: _____	Date: _____

Skill: **Self-Determination and No CPR Requests**

Steps	Completed	Comments
CPR 1. The resident must be informed he/she may initiate an advance directive upon admission. An *advance directive* may be either a *living will*, a *durable power of attorney for healthcare*, or both. Some states have additional, state-specific directives available.		
2. CPR will be attempted for all residents unless there is a "No CPR" order written by the physician on the physician's order sheet and documentation from the resident, family, or responsible party of this request.		
3. A "No CPR" request may be reversed at any time when the request is given in writing by the resident, family, or responsible party.		
4. If CPR is initiated, 911 will be dialed to summon emergency medical aid. Personnel will continue CPR until care is transferred to ambulance personnel.		
5. Once CPR is initiated, it will not be stopped unless a present physician orders it to be stopped.		
Self-Determination 1. Upon admission, residents will be given the option of filling out an advanced directive to inform the facility of their requests for care pertaining to various life sustaining procedures.		
2. If the resident informs the facility in writing of a request for no CPR or no feeding tubes, etc., the facility will contact the attending physician and inform him or her the request.		
3. The attending physician will then give a written order to comply with the resident's request.		
4. The facility will then comply with the resident's request.		

Self-assessment	Evaluation/ validation methods	Levels	Type of validation	Comments
❏ Experienced ❏ Need practice ❏ Never done ❏ Not applicable (based on scope of practice)	❏ Verbal ❏ Demonstration/ observation ❏ Practical exercise ❏ Interactive class	❏ Beginner ❏ Intermediate ❏ Expert	❏ Orientation ❏ Annual ❏ Other _____	

Employee signature   **Observer signature**

Name: _____ Date: _____

Skill: **Self-Administration of Medications**

Steps	Completed	Comments
1. The physician must approve and an order will be taken to have the medication kept at the bedside.		
2. The interdisciplinary team, which will include an RN will assess the safety of the resident self-administering his or her own medication.		
3. If the interdisciplinary team determines the resident as safe to self-administer his or her medication, the medication shall be given to the resident.		

Self-assessment	Evaluation/ validation methods	Levels	Type of validation	Comments
❏ Experienced ❏ Need practice ❏ Never done ❏ Not applicable (based on scope of practice)	❏ Verbal ❏ Demonstration/ observation ❏ Practical exercise ❏ Interactive class	❏ Beginner ❏ Intermediate ❏ Expert	❏ Orientation ❏ Annual ❏ Other _____	

_____
Employee signature

_____
Observer signature

Name: _____ Date: _____

Skill: **Care of the Resident Who Has Public Displays of Sexual Behaviors**

Steps	Completed	Comments
1. Always explain the reasons and procedures to the resident.		
2. Always approach the resident calmly and unhurriedly. Speak in a calm voice.		
3. Assist the resident to a private area or by pulling the privacy curtain.		
4. Attempt to refocus behavior to something positive when the resident is exhibiting inappropriate behavior.		
5. If appropriate, stop giving care when the resident is inappropriate and try later.		
6. Encourage activities of the resident's choice and preference.		
7. Explain why sexual relationships are special and it is better if they are done in private.		
8. Encourage the resident to discuss interests or concerns.		
9. Involve the family in the care if possible or available.		
10. Notify the physician if the behavior interferes with functioning.		

Self-assessment	Evaluation/ validation methods	Levels	Type of validation	Comments
❏ Experienced ❏ Need practice ❏ Never done ❏ Not applicable (based on scope of practice)	❏ Verbal ❏ Demonstration/ observation ❏ Practical exercise ❏ Interactive class	❏ Beginner ❏ Intermediate ❏ Expert	❏ Orientation ❏ Annual ❏ Other _____	

_____ _____
Employee signature   **Observer signature**

Name: _____   Date: _____

Skill: **Shampoo**

Steps	Completed	Comments
1. Explain the reason and procedure to the resident.		
2. Unless the resident has the hair done by the hair dresser, wash the hair during the shower at least once a week. Give the resident a dry washcloth to cover the eyes during the shampoo and rinsing.		
3. Report any scaly skin, open areas, or other irritation promptly.		

Self-assessment	Evaluation/ validation methods	Levels	Type of validation	Comments
❑ Experienced ❑ Need practice ❑ Never done ❑ Not applicable (based on scope of practice)	❑ Verbal ❑ Demonstration/ observation ❑ Practical exercise ❑ Interactive class	❑ Beginner ❑ Intermediate ❑ Expert	❑ Orientation ❑ Annual ❑ Other _____	

_____   _____
Employee signature   **Observer signature**

Name: _____ Date: _____

Skill: **Shower**

Steps	Completed	Comments
1. Explain the purpose and procedure to the resident.		
2. Get the shower chair, soap, towel, washcloth, and clean clothes. Clean shower area and shower chair.		
3. Pull the curtain and transfer the resident to the shower chair. Lock the wheels. Ensure that the resident is not exposed.		
4. Adjust the water spray and temperature. Check the temperature on your forearm before using to ensure it is not too hot. Keep the spray of warm water on at least one area of the resident's body during the entire procedure to prevent chilling.		
5. Undress the resident. Wrap the resident with a bath blanket. Cover the resident's genitalia with a towel for modesty. Remove the bath blanket when you are ready to begin bathing.		
6. Encourage the resident to wash as much as possible independently.		
7. Assist the resident in washing hard-to-reach areas and shampooing the hair. If you wash the resident's hair, placing cotton in the ears will keep them free from water in case the spray is misdirected. Bring an extra towel to wrap the head after rinsing the shampoo.		
8. Wrap the resident with the dry bath blanket when you turn the water off. Dry the resident promptly and dress.		
9. Monitor for and report red or open areas or bruises.		
10. Discard used clothes and linen in the appropriate barrels. After the resident is cared for, return to clean and disinfect the shower and shower chair.		
11. Always hang the hand-held shower spray on the hook when not in use. To prevent contamination, it should never touch the floor.		

Self-assessment	Evaluation/ validation methods	Levels	Type of validation	Comments
❑ Experienced ❑ Need practice ❑ Never done ❑ Not applicable (based on scope of practice)	❑ Verbal ❑ Demonstration/ observation ❑ Practical exercise ❑ Interactive class	❑ Beginner ❑ Intermediate ❑ Expert	❑ Orientation ❑ Annual ❑ Other _____	

_____
Employee signature

_____
Observer signature

 Competency Management in Long-Term Care

Name: _____ Date: _____

Skill: **Arteriovenous Shunt Care**

Steps	Completed	Comments
1. Explain the reason and procedure to the resident.		
2. Wash your hands and pull the curtain.		
3. Put on your gloves.		
4. Remove the old dressing.		
5. Observe the shunt for edema, redness, tenderness, or drainage. If found, report immediately to the physician.		
6. Place your fingertips lightly on the shunt to feel the bruit (pulsation of blood). Report lack of the bruit immediately to the physician.		
7. Follow the physician's orders for cleaning the shunt.		
8. Change your gloves.		
9. Apply a new dressing. Ensure that it isn't too tight.		
10. Remove your gloves.		
11. Wash your hands.		

Self-assessment	Evaluation/ validation methods	Levels	Type of validation	Comments
❏ Experienced ❏ Need practice ❏ Never done ❏ Not applicable (based on scope of practice)	❏ Verbal ❏ Demonstration/ observation ❏ Practical exercise ❏ Interactive class	❏ Beginner ❏ Intermediate ❏ Expert	❏ Orientation ❏ Annual ❏ Other _____	

_____
Employee signature

_____
Observer signature

Name: _____ Date: _____

Skill: **Monitoring the Side Effects for Psychosocial Medications**

Steps	Completed	Comments
1. Monitor the resident for possible side effects.		
2. Report any side effects promptly to the attending physician or psychiatrist.		
3. Hold the medication and monitor the vital signs until the physician is notified if the side effects are lethargy or excessive drowsiness.		

Self-assessment	Evaluation/ validation methods	Levels	Type of validation	Comments
❏ Experienced ❏ Need practice ❏ Never done ❏ Not applicable (based on scope of practice)	❏ Verbal ❏ Demonstration/ observation ❏ Practical exercise ❏ Interactive class	❏ Beginner ❏ Intermediate ❏ Expert	❏ Orientation ❏ Annual ❏ Other _____	

_____
Employee signature

_____
Observer signature

Name: _____ Date: _____

Skill: **Sitz Bath**

Steps	Completed	Comments
1. Explain the reason and procedure to the resident.		
2. Clean and disinfect the tub, if necessary. Ask the resident if she needs to void before beginning. Assist if necessary.		
3. Fill the tub or sitz bath basin one-third to one-half full of warm water so the perineum will be completely immersed. Fill the irrigation bag with 105° F to 110° F water. (Water will cool before use.) Hang the solution on the towel bar or an IV pole.		
4. Insert the tubing through the entry hole at the front of the plastic bowl. Pull the tubing to the inside and secure by snapping into the channel in the center bottom of the bowl. Be sure the small hole at the end of the tubing faces upward.		
5. Assist the resident in positioning. Support the feet if they do not reach the floor. Wrap a bath blanket around the resident's shoulders. Drape a second bath blanket across the lap. Offer to place the over-bed table in front of the resident, if desired for additional support.		
6. Open the clamp to initiate the flow of solution. Show the resident how to regulate the flow, if he or she is able. (If the resident is confused, remain in the room during the procedure and assist as needed.) Refill the irrigation bag if necessary.		
7. Have the resident sit in water for 15 to 20 minutes, or as ordered by the physician.		
8. Assist the resident to use the handrail to stand. Monitor for dizziness, weakness, feeling faint, or nauseated.		
9. Assist with drying, if necessary.		
10. Apply a clean dressing or peri pad, if needed.		
11. Assist the resident to dress and return to his or her room.		
12. Position the resident for comfort and make sure the call signal and needed personal items are within reach.		
13. Return to the bathroom and wash, disinfect, and dry the sitz tub.		
14. Store the disposable sitz tub for reuse.		

Self-assessment	Evaluation/ validation methods	Levels	Type of validation	Comments
❏ Experienced ❏ Need practice ❏ Never done ❏ Not applicable (based on scope of practice)	❏ Verbal ❏ Demonstration/ observation ❏ Practical exercise ❏ Interactive class	❏ Beginner ❏ Intermediate ❏ Expert	❏ Orientation ❏ Annual ❏ Other _____	

_____   _____
Employee signature   **Observer signature**

Name: _____   Date: _____

Skill: **Foley Catheter Urine Specimen Collection**

Steps	Completed	Comments
1. Explain the reason and procedure to the resident. Prepare the label for the specimen. Obtain a sterile specimen cup with lid and plastic transport bag.		
2. Wash your hands and pull the curtain.		
3. Put on your gloves.		
4. Clamp the catheter below the collection port for 15 to 20 minutes.		
5. Remove the lid for the specimen cup and place it on the table with the clean inside facing up.		
6. Wipe the collection port well with an alcohol pad. Allow to dry.		
7. Remove the cap to the needle and rotate the syringe so the bevel is facing up. Insert the needle into the collection port at a 30- to 45-degree angle.		
8. Gently pull back on the plunger to withdraw the sample. Collect at least 10 ml, or as required by the lab.		
9. Remove the needle. Depress the plunger gently to transfer the specimen into the sterile cup without splashing.		
10. Cap the specimen cup and place on paper towel. Discard the syringe into the sharps' container.		
11. Remove the clamp from the catheter. Remove your gloves.		
12. Assist the resident with dressing and handwashing, as needed.		
13. Position the resident for comfort. Be sure he or she has the call signal and needed personal items within reach.		
14. Wash your hands.		
15. Label the specimen, place it into a transport bag with the requisition affixed. Place in the specimen refrigerator.		
16. Wash your hands.		

Self-assessment	Evaluation/ validation methods	Levels	Type of validation	Comments
❑ Experienced ❑ Need practice ❑ Never done ❑ Not applicable (based on scope of practice)	❑ Verbal ❑ Demonstration/ observation ❑ Practical exercise ❑ Interactive class	❑ Beginner ❑ Intermediate ❑ Expert	❑ Orientation ❑ Annual ❑ Other _____ _____	

_____   _____
Employee signature   **Observer signature**

Name: _____ Date: _____

Skill: **Mid-Stream Urine Specimen Collection**

Steps	Completed	Comments
1. Explain the reason and procedure to the resident. Prepare a label for the specimen container and obtain a sterile specimen cup with lid and a plastic transport bag.		
2. If the resident is ambulatory, assist him or her to the bathroom. If non-ambulatory, pull the curtain and place the resident on the bedpan.		
3. Put on your gloves.		
4. Assist the resident in washing off genitalia. For female residents, wash from front to back.		
5. After the resident voided a small amount, place the collection container in flow of urine and collect a sample. After you have obtained 30 ml to 50 ml, remove the cup and have the resident finish emptying the bladder. Cap the specimen cup and place it on a paper towel.		
6. Remove your gloves.		
7. Assist the resident with handwashing and dressing, if needed.		
8. Position the resident for comfort.		
9. Label the specimen, place in transport bag, and attach requisition. Place in the specimen refrigerator for later pickup.		
10. Wash your hands.		

Self-assessment	Evaluation/ validation methods	Levels	Type of validation	Comments
❏ Experienced ❏ Need practice ❏ Never done ❏ Not applicable (based on scope of practice)	❏ Verbal ❏ Demonstration/ observation ❏ Practical exercise ❏ Interactive class	❏ Beginner ❏ Intermediate ❏ Expert	❏ Orientation ❏ Annual ❏ Other _____	

_____
Employee signature

_____
Observer signature

Name: _____ Date: _____

Skill: **Routine Urine Specimen Collection**

Steps	Completed	Comments
1. Explain the reason and procedure to the resident. Prepare a label for the specimen container and obtain a non-sterile specimen cup with lid and a plastic transport bag.		
2. If the resident is ambulatory, assist him or her to the bathroom. If non-ambulatory, pull the curtain and place resident on a clean bedpan.		
3. Put on your gloves.		
4. Assist the resident in washing off genitalia. For female residents, wash from front to back.		
5. Have the resident void in the bedpan or the urine collection container. Instruct the resident not to drop toilet tissue into the specimen. Provide a plastic bag for disposal, if necessary. If voiding in the bedpan, pour a sample of the urine into the container. Cap the specimen cup and place on paper towel.		
6. Remove your gloves.		
7. Assist the resident with handwashing and dressing, if needed.		
8. Position the resident for comfort.		
9. Label the specimen, place in transport bag, and attach requisition. Place in the specimen refrigerator for later pickup.		
10. Wash your hands.		

Self-assessment	Evaluation/ validation methods	Levels	Type of validation	Comments
❏ Experienced ❏ Need practice ❏ Never done ❏ Not applicable (based on scope of practice)	❏ Verbal ❏ Demonstration/ observation ❏ Practical exercise ❏ Interactive class	❏ Beginner ❏ Intermediate ❏ Expert	❏ Orientation ❏ Annual ❏ Other _____	

_____
Employee signature

_____
Observer signature

Name: _____ Date: _____

Skill: **Sputum Specimen Collection**

Steps	Completed	Comments
1. Explain the reason and procedure to the resident.		
2. Wash your hands, put on gloves, and pull the curtain.		
3. Assist the resident in rinsing out his or her mouth with water.		
4. Ask the resident to take several deep breaths, then cough deeply to bring up a sputum specimen. Obtain 15 ml, if possible.		
5. Ask the resident to expectorate into the specimen container. Cap the container. Handle the container with gloves and wipe the outside surface with disinfectant solution.		
6. Affix the label to the container after disinfecting. Place the specimen container in a plastic transport bag.		
7. Remove and discard gloves.		
8. Assist the resident to a position of comfort and safety. Make sure the call signal and needed personal items are within reach.		
9. Wash your hands.		
10. Transport the specimen to the lab immediately.		

Self-assessment	Evaluation/ validation methods	Levels	Type of validation	Comments
❏ Experienced ❏ Need practice ❏ Never done ❏ Not applicable (based on scope of practice)	❏ Verbal ❏ Demonstration/ observation ❏ Practical exercise ❏ Interactive class	❏ Beginner ❏ Intermediate ❏ Expert	❏ Orientation ❏ Annual ❏ Other _____	

_____
Employee signature

_____
Observer signature

| Name: _____ | Date: _____ |

Skill: **Stool Specimen Collection**

Steps	Completed	Comments
1. Obtain a non-sterile specimen cup with a lid and a plastic transport bag. Prepare a label for the container. Obtain a plastic bag or other covered container for waste.		
2. Explain the reason and procedure to the resident. Ask the resident to inform you when he or she is going to have a bowel movement.		
3. Put on your gloves.		
4. Pull the curtain and place the resident on a sanitized bedpan or assist to the bathroom. Place a specimen collection container ("specimen hat") under the toilet seat. Provide a separate container for urination, if necessary. Ask the resident not to void in the stool specimen collection device, or ask the resident to wait to urinate until you have removed the stool specimen.		
5. After the resident has had the bowel movement, remove and cover the bedpan. Assist with cleaning, handwashing, and dressing.		
6. Place the specimen collection container on a paper towel. Open the lid and put it aside, with the clean inner side facing up.		
7. With the tongue blade, remove feces from the collection device and transfer to the specimen container. Collect approximately two to four tablespoons. Taking a small sample from each part of the stool is best. Collect any substance or colored area that appears abnormal. Discard the tongue blade in a plastic bag or other designated container.		
8. Cap the container. Handle the container with gloves and wipe the outside surface with disinfectant solution.		
9. Affix the label to the container after disinfecting. Place the specimen container in a plastic transport bag.		
10. Remove and discard gloves.		

   Competency Management in Long-Term Care

11. Assist the resident to a position of comfort and safety. Make sure the call signal and needed personal items are within reach.		
12. Wash your hands.		
13. Discard the plastic bag containing the waste in the biohazardous waste container when leaving the room.		
14. Transport the specimen to the laboratory as soon as possible after collection.		

Self-assessment	Evaluation/ validation methods	Levels	Type of validation	Comments
❏ Experienced ❏ Need practice ❏ Never done ❏ Not applicable (based on scope of practice)	❏ Verbal ❏ Demonstration/ observation ❏ Practical exercise ❏ Interactive class	❏ Beginner ❏ Intermediate ❏ Expert	❏ Orientation ❏ Annual ❏ Other _____	

_____
Employee signature

_____
Observer signature

Name: _____ Date: _____

Skill: **Staple Removal**

Steps	Completed	Comments
Sutures and staples are usually removed in 7 to 10 days. Leaving them longer increases the risk of infection. Assess the wound and inform the physician of its appearance and healing progress. Obtain an order for staple removal.		
1. Explain the reason and procedure to the resident. Inform the resident that he or she may feel slight discomfort, pulling, and/or pinching, but that the procedure is not painful.		
2. Wash your hands and pull the curtain.		
3. Establish a clean work area and put on your gloves.		
4. Remove the dressing and discard in a plastic bag.		
5. Cleanse the suture line with normal saline or pH neutral wound cleanser. Remove your gloves and discard them in the plastic bag.		
6. Wash your hands or use alcohol-based hand cleaner.		
7. Apply sterile gloves.		
8. Slide the staple removal device under the first staple. Squeeze the handles.		
9. Gently lift the staple out. Placed used staples on a gauze pad.		
10. Repeat this procedure to remove every other staple. Assess the skin to be sure the suture line is not separating. After you have finished removing every other staple, apply a Steri-Strip® or Butterfly® to the area where each staple was removed.		
11. Remove the remaining staples. Apply a Steri-Strip® or Butterfly® to each area.		
12. Cleanse the wound with normal saline or pH neutral wound cleanser, and dress the wound.		
13. Discard the used staples, gauze pad, soiled dressing, and other contaminated supplies in a plastic bag.		

 Competency Management in Long-Term Care

14. Remove your gloves and discard in plastic bag. Discard the plastic bag containing the waste in the biohazardous waste container when leaving the room.		
15. Assist the resident to a position of comfort and safety. Make sure the call signal and needed personal items are within reach.		
16. Document the procedure and your observations.		

Self-assessment	Evaluation/ validation methods	Levels	Type of validation	Comments
❑ Experienced ❑ Need practice ❑ Never done ❑ Not applicable (based on scope of practice)	❑ Verbal ❑ Demonstration/ observation ❑ Practical exercise ❑ Interactive class	❑ Beginner ❑ Intermediate ❑ Expert	❑ Orientation ❑ Annual ❑ Other _____	

_____
Employee signature

_____
Observer signature

Name: _____	Date: _____	

Skill: Suctioning

Steps	Completed	Comments
1. Explain the reason and procedure to the resident.		
2. Wash your hands and pull the curtain.		
3. Provide supplemental oxygen before suctioning, if needed, or if this is your facility policy. Remember, the resident cannot breathe during suctioning.		
4. Pour sterile water into a sterile tray or basin.		
5. Attach the connecting tubing to the suction regulator, and turn the suction on. Place one finger over the distal end of the tubing to check the suction pressure while the tube is blocked.		
6. Open the sterile package for the suction catheter. Attach the connecting tubing to the proximal catheter. Expose only the connecting, keeping the distal end covered inside the wrapper.		
7. Apply sterile gloves. Keep the glove on your dominant hand sterile, and use the nondominant hand to touch non-sterile items. Use the nondominant hand to open and close the thumb valve while controlling the catheter with your other hand.		
8. Connect the catheter to the connecting tubing with your sterile hand.		
9. Carefully insert the catheter 3 to 4 inches into one side of the resident's mouth, or until you reach the pool of secretions, without applying suction.		
10. Initiate suctioning by covering the thumb valve, or opening the catheter and suctioning the secretions. Move the catheter to both sides of the mouth in a continuous rotating motion.		
11. Suction for no longer than 10 seconds, including the time it takes to withdraw the catheter.		
12. Clear the tube by suctioning sterile water while allowing the resident to recover and breathe normally. If you will be reinserting the catheter, wrap it around your dominant hand, leaving the distal end free, to prevent contamination.		

13. Repeat the suctioning until gurgling or bubbling stops and the resident's respirations are silent.		
14. Remove your gloves.		
15. Position the resident for comfort and safety. Make sure the call signal and needed personal items are within reach.		
16. Wash your hands.		
17. Document the procedure and your observations.		

Self-assessment	Evaluation/ validation methods	Levels	Type of validation	Comments
❏ Experienced ❏ Need practice ❏ Never done ❏ Not applicable (based on scope of practice)	❏ Verbal ❏ Demonstration/ observation ❏ Practical exercise ❏ Interactive class	❏ Beginner ❏ Intermediate ❏ Expert	❏ Orientation ❏ Annual ❏ Other _____	

_____
Employee signature

_____
Observer signature

Name:	Date:

Skill: Rectal Suppository Administration

Steps	Completed	Comments
1. Explain the reason and procedure to the resident.		
2. Provide privacy by pulling the curtain.		
3. Wash your hands and apply gloves.		
4. Position the resident in the left Sims' position.		
5. Remove the wrapper and lubricate the suppository with water-soluble lubricant.		
6. Separate the buttocks. Instruct the resident to take a deep breath.		
7. Insert suppository gently through the anal opening, directing it along the rectal wall toward umbilicus, approximately 2 inches, using the index finger.		
8. Instruct the resident to retain the suppository for 20 minutes, if able. Make sure that the bedpan is available.		
9. Wipe off excess lubricant with toilet paper.		
10. Remove gloves and discard in plastic bag or other appropriate container.		
11. Position the resident for comfort with the call light available. Respond promptly if the resident calls.		
12. Wash your hands.		

Self-assessment	Evaluation/ validation methods	Levels	Type of validation	Comments
❑ Experienced ❑ Need practice ❑ Never done ❑ Not applicable (based on scope of practice)	❑ Verbal ❑ Demonstration/ observation ❑ Practical exercise ❑ Interactive class	❑ Beginner ❑ Intermediate ❑ Expert	❑ Orientation ❑ Annual ❑ Other _____	

_____
Employee signature

_____
Observer signature

Name: _____ Date: _____

Skill: **Vaginal Suppository Administration**

Steps	Completed	Comments
1. Explain the reason and procedure to the resident.		
2. Wash hands and apply gloves. Provide privacy by pulling the curtain.		
3. Position the resident on her back with legs spread and perineum exposed. Cover with bath blanket for modesty and dignity.		
4. Remove the wrapper and lubricate the suppository, if necessary.		
5. Separate the labia and insert the suppository approximately 2 inches upward and backward into the vagina.		
6. Apply a sanitary napkin.		
7. Remove gloves and discard in plastic bag, or according to facility policy.		
8. Have the resident remain in a recumbent position for 30 minutes, then assist with positioning or mobility as desired or needed.		
9. Position the resident for comfort and safety with the call light and needed personal items within reach. Return promptly if the resident signals.		
10. Wash your hands.		

Self-assessment	Evaluation/ validation methods	Levels	Type of validation	Comments
❏ Experienced ❏ Need practice ❏ Never done ❏ Not applicable (based on scope of practice)	❏ Verbal ❏ Demonstration/ observation ❏ Practical exercise ❏ Interactive class	❏ Beginner ❏ Intermediate ❏ Expert	❏ Orientation ❏ Annual ❏ Other _____	

_____
Employee signature

_____
Observer signature

Name: _____	Date: _____	

Skill: **Suture Removal**

Steps	Completed	Comments
Sutures and staples are usually removed in 7 to 10 days. Leaving them longer increases the risk of infection. Assess the wound and inform the physician of its appearance and healing progress. Obtain an order for staple removal.		
1. Explain the reason and procedure to the resident. Inform the resident that he or she may feel slight discomfort, pulling, and/or pinching, but that the procedure is not painful.		
2. Wash your hands and pull the curtain.		
3. Establish a sterile work area and put on your gloves. Remove the dressing and discard in a plastic bag.		
4. Remove the dressing and cleanse the suture line with normal saline or pH neutral wound cleanser. Remove your gloves and discard them in the plastic bag.		
5. Wash your hands or use alcohol-based hand cleaner.		
6. Apply sterile gloves.		
7. Use the forceps to grasp the knot of the first suture.		
8. Gently raise the suture off the skin and cut one end.		
9. Gently pull the suture out while holding the knotted end with the forceps. Discard on gauze sponge. Discard all the sutures and the pad in the plastic bag after all sutures are removed.		
10. Continue by removing every other suture by lifting the suture up, away from the skin, with the tweezers. Cut the suture close to the skin.		
11. With the tweezers, lift the suture up by the knot, and pull it through the skin in one piece.		
12. Assess the skin to be sure the suture line is not separating. After you have finished removing every other suture, apply a Steri-Strip® or Butterfly® to the area where each suture was removed.		
13. Remove the remaining sutures. Apply a Steri-Strip® or Butterfly® to each area.		
14. Cleanse the wound with normal saline or pH neutral wound cleanser, and dress the wound.		

15. Discard the used sutures, gauze pad, soiled dressing, and other contaminated supplies in a plastic bag.		
16. Remove your gloves and discard in plastic bag. Discard the plastic bag containing the waste in the biohazardous waste container when leaving the room.		
17. Assist the resident to a position of comfort and safety. Make sure the call signal and needed personal items are within reach.		
18. Wash your hands or use alcohol-based hand cleanser.		
19. Document the procedure and your observations.		

Self-assessment	Evaluation/ validation methods	Levels	Type of validation	Comments
❏ Experienced ❏ Need practice ❏ Never done ❏ Not applicable (based on scope of practice)	❏ Verbal ❏ Demonstration/ observation ❏ Practical exercise ❏ Interactive class	❏ Beginner ❏ Intermediate ❏ Expert	❏ Orientation ❏ Annual ❏ Other _____	

_____
Employee signature

_____
Observer signature

Name: _____	Date: _____	

Skill: Syringe Feeding

Steps	Completed	Comments
1. Explain the reason and procedure to the resident.		
2. Wash your hands.		
3. Position the resident in the semi-Fowler's or Fowler's position, as tolerated. The head and shoulders should be elevated at least 30 degrees. Make sure the neck is in the neutral position, so it is not bent back or flexed forward. (Either of these increases the risk of complications.)		
4. Identify the resident and check the tray card for the correct name and diet. Check the tray for correct food items, condiments, and utensils (if needed). Review any special feeding instructions provided by the speech therapist, if applicable.		
5. Place the meal tray on the overbed table and describe the food.		
6. Place a napkin or clothing protector under resident's chin and across the chest.		
7. Ask resident what food is preferred.		
8. Fill the syringe with between 15 ml and 30 ml of liquefied blenderized food.		
9. Insert the tip of the syringe into the resident's mouth. If he or she has had a stroke, direct it towards the back of the cheek on the dominant side.		
10. Slowly push the plunger.		
11. Allow the resident enough time to swallow. Provide verbal cues, if indicated. Offer fluids as the resident wishes. Be observant for coughing or signs and symptoms of swallowing difficulty. If observed, stop feeding and immediately alert the nurse.		
12. Repeat steps 4–7 until the resident has consumed 100% of the meal, or as much as desired. Avoid forcing the resident to eat.		
13. Wipe resident's mouth, as needed.		
14. Remove the clothing protector.		
15. Wash the resident's face and hands.		

16. Leave the head of the bed elevated for 60 minutes, or according to facility policy.		
17. Document fluid intake and output, if appropriate.		
18. Wash your hands.		
19. Document total meal intake according to facility policy.		

Self-assessment	Evaluation/ validation methods	Levels	Type of validation	Comments
❏ Experienced ❏ Need practice ❏ Never done ❏ Not applicable (based on scope of practice)	❏ Verbal ❏ Demonstration/ observation ❏ Practical exercise ❏ Interactive class	❏ Beginner ❏ Intermediate ❏ Expert	❏ Orientation ❏ Annual ❏ Other _____	

_____
Employee signature

_____
Observer signature

| Name: _____ | Date: _____ |

Skill: **TED Hose**

Steps	Completed	Comments
1. Explain the reason and procedure to the resident.		
2. Wash your hands and pull the curtain.		
3. Apply hosiery before the resident gets out of bed in the morning.		
4. Check the skin on the leg prior to applying the stockings for redness, warmth, swelling, excessive dryness, or open areas. Notify nurse if abnormalities present. Continue procedure only if instructed.		
5. Grasp the center of the heel pocket and turn stocking inside out to the heel area. Position the stocking over the foot and heel. Center the heel in the heel pocket.		
6. Begin pulling the body of the stocking around the ankle and calf.		
7. Gently snap the fabric up around the ankle to ensure a tight fit and eliminate gaps.		
8. Continue to apply the stocking over the leg until the full length of the hose is on the leg.		
9. Smooth the stockings to remove any wrinkles. Ensure that the stocking is not bunched up or folded over.		
10. Adjust the foot section for fabric smoothness and toe comfort by tugging on the top section.		
11. Check the skin every four hours or as instructed. Look through and pull back the inspection hole in the end to ensure the toes are warm and of normal color, and circulation is adequate.		
12. Remove the stockings as ordered (usually at bedtime, but at least once daily) and monitor skin closely. Always remove stockings for bathing.		
13. Monitor the skin, swelling, warmth or coolness of the extremity, abnormal color, or discomfort.		

Self-assessment	Evaluation/ validation methods	Levels	Type of validation	Comments
❑ Experienced ❑ Need practice ❑ Never done ❑ Not applicable (based on scope of practice)	❑ Verbal ❑ Demonstration/ observation ❑ Practical exercise ❑ Interactive class	❑ Beginner ❑ Intermediate ❑ Expert	❑ Orientation ❑ Annual ❑ Other _____	

_____
Employee signature

_____
Observer signature

Name: _____ Date: _____

Skill: **Oral Temperature**

Steps	Completed	Comments
1. Explain the reason and procedure to the resident.		
2. Wash your hands.		
3. Rinse disinfectant off the thermometer with cool water and dry. Shake down the thermometer until the mercury is below 95° F.		
4. Insert the thermometer into a disposable sheath.		
5. Insert the bulb end of the thermometer under the resident's tongue as far back as possible.		
6. Ask the resident to keep his or her mouth closed.		
7. Remove after three minutes. Remove and discard sheath.		
8. Hold the thermometer at eye level. Rotate until the mercury (or alcohol) line appears. Accurately read and record the temperature.		
9. Shake down the thermometer, and clean and store according to facility policy.		
10. Wash your hands.		
11. Inform the charge nurse of an oral reading below 96° F or above 99° F.		

Self-assessment	Evaluation/ validation methods	Levels	Type of validation	Comments
❏ Experienced ❏ Need practice ❏ Never done ❏ Not applicable (based on scope of practice)	❏ Verbal ❏ Demonstration/ observation ❏ Practical exercise ❏ Interactive class	❏ Beginner ❏ Intermediate ❏ Expert	❏ Orientation ❏ Annual ❏ Other _____	

_____
Employee signature

_____
Observer signature

Name: _____ Date: _____

Skill: **Rectal Temperature**

Steps	Completed	Comments
1. Explain the reason and procedure to the resident.		
2. Wash your hands.		
3. Rinse disinfectant off the thermometer with cool water and dry. Shake down the thermometer until the mercury is below 95° F.		
4. Insert the thermometer into a disposable sheath.		
5. Place a small amount of lubricant on a tissue or paper towel. Use the tissue to lubricate the bulb of the thermometer, if needed. (Some plastic sheaths are pre-lubricated).		
6. Position the resident on his or her side.		
7. Separate the buttocks.		
8. Insert the thermometer into the rectum approximately 1 inch.		
9. Hold the thermometer in place at least three minutes.		
10. Remove the thermometer. Hold the thermometer at eye level and read the mercury column. Note the reading.		
11. Place the thermometer in container for used thermometers or disinfect according to facility policy.		
12. Remove gloves and discard according to facility policy.		
13. Record the temperature reading.		
14. Wash your hands.		

Self-assessment	Evaluation/ validation methods	Levels	Type of validation	Comments
❏ Experienced ❏ Need practice ❏ Never done ❏ Not applicable (based on scope of practice)	❏ Verbal ❏ Demonstration/ observation ❏ Practical exercise ❏ Interactive class	❏ Beginner ❏ Intermediate ❏ Expert	❏ Orientation ❏ Annual ❏ Other _____	

Employee signature _____ **Observer signature** _____

Name: _____ Date: _____

Skill: **Transferring a Resident Out of the Facility**

Steps	Completed	Comments
1. Obtain a physician's order for transfer or discharge. Clarify whether medications should be sent with the resident.		
2. Explain the reason and procedure to the resident. If the resident is discharging to home, review the discharge plan of care with the resident and/or responsible party and ensure they understand it.		
3. Complete the inter-facility transfer form when sending the resident to the acute hospital. Complete the Discharge summary when sending the resident home or to another non-acute care facility. When sending the resident to another facility, send a copy of the most recent History and Physical, copy of pertinent lab or X-ray results, MDS, care plan, discharge plan of care, and the most recent physician's orders.		
4. Notify the family and/or surrogate decision-maker of the reason and location.		
5. Collect the resident's belongings.		
6. Check the belongings against the personal inventory or clothing list to ensure that the resident has all belongings.		
7. Complete and have the resident or responsible party sign the clothing inventory.		
8. Assist with packing, if necessary.		
9. Assist the resident to dress, if necessary.		
10. Assist the resident to transfer to the wheelchair or stretcher, as appropriate. Notify the ambulance company, if needed.		
11. Notify the emergency room of the impending transfer and reason, if appropriate.		
12. Transfer the resident into a wheelchair or monitor/assist the transfer of the resident onto the gurney.		
13. Transport the resident to the car. Assist the resident into the car.		
14. Say goodbye to the resident.		
15. Document the above in the nurses' notes.		

Self-assessment	Evaluation/ validation methods	Levels	Type of validation	Comments
❏ Experienced ❏ Need practice ❏ Never done ❏ Not applicable (based on scope of practice)	❏ Verbal ❏ Demonstration/ observation ❏ Practical exercise ❏ Interactive class	❏ Beginner ❏ Intermediate ❏ Expert	❏ Orientation ❏ Annual ❏ Other _____	

_____   _____
Employee signature   **Observer signature**

Name:	Date:

Skill: Serving Meals

Steps	Completed	Comments
1. Wash your hands.		
2. Assist residents with toileting and handwashing before meals.		
3. Ensure that the resident who wears dentures has them in.		
4. If necessary, provide protection for the resident's clothing.		
5. Serve one table at a time. Residents should not have to watch others eat while waiting for their own food. Serve slow eaters first, if possible.		
6. If a closed food cart is used, close the door after removing each tray. This will maintain food temperature and prevent contamination.		
7. Identify each resident. Check the diet card against the items on the tray for accuracy and food preferences.		
8. Replace missing food items, if needed.		
9. Keep food covered during transportation to maintain temperature and prevent contamination.		
10. Remove food from the tray and place on the table in front of the resident, if this is your facility policy. If not, place the tray in front of the resident.		
11. Prepare the meal, if necessary, by removing covers, opening packages and wrappers, such as foil and plastic, peeling food such as fruit, opening milk and yogurt cartons, providing straws, cutting meat, buttering bread, stirring sugar or lemon into beverages, if needed, and putting condiments on food.		
12. Position the plate with the main course closest to the resident.		
13. Assist the resident with the napkin, if needed.		
14. Provide adaptive eating devices, if used.		
15. Leave trays on the food cart until you are ready to feed the residents. Do not put a tray in front of a resident who must be spoon fed until you are available to assist with the meal.		

16. Serve all clean trays before returning used trays to the food cart. Do not return used trays if uneaten food remains on the cart.		
17. If you stop serving trays to assist a resident, wash your hands (or use alcohol hand cleaner) before continuing.		
18. If the resident needs to be fed, slowly offer small portions at a time.		
19. If the resident can eat independently, you may leave the resident and assist others. Make sure that the call light is within reach.		
20. Monitor residents frequently during meal time. Offer to replace or reheat food that has become cold. Honor requests for substitutes and extra portions, if allowed on diet. Fluids are particularly important. Always offer beverage refills.		
21. After removing the tray, ensure that the resident and the area are clean and free of food particles.		
22. Record the residents' meal intake by percentage consumed. Report refused meals promptly to the charge nurse.		

Self-assessment	Evaluation/ validation methods	Levels	Type of validation	Comments
❏ Experienced ❏ Need practice ❏ Never done ❏ Not applicable (based on scope of practice)	❏ Verbal ❏ Demonstration/ observation ❏ Practical exercise ❏ Interactive class	❏ Beginner ❏ Intermediate ❏ Expert	❏ Orientation ❏ Annual ❏ Other _____	

_____   _____
Employee signature   **Observer signature**

Name: _____ Date: _____

Skill: **Assisting with the Urinal**

Steps	Completed	Comments
1. Explain the reason and procedure to the resident. Wash your hands.		
2. Screen the resident.		
3. If the resident is able to use the urinal independently, place a clean urinal within reach. Ensure that the call light is available and answered promptly.		
4. If the resident needs assistance, apply gloves. Place the urinal between his legs. Position the penis in the urinal. Ensure that there is no pressure from the urinal between his legs. Do not leave the urinal in place for a prolonged period of time.		
5. When the resident has finished, remove and cover the urinal.		
6. Take urinal to bathroom, check urine for color, odor, amount, clarity, and character and report unusual findings to the nurse.		
7. Discard urine, sanitize, and return the urinal to its designated storage area.		
8. Provide the resident with a washcloth to wash his hands.		
9. Record the output if on intake and output monitoring.		
10. Wash your hands.		

Self-assessment	Evaluation/ validation methods	Levels	Type of validation	Comments
❏ Experienced ❏ Need practice ❏ Never done ❏ Not applicable (based on scope of practice)	❏ Verbal ❏ Demonstration/ observation ❏ Practical exercise ❏ Interactive class	❏ Beginner ❏ Intermediate ❏ Expert	❏ Orientation ❏ Annual ❏ Other _____	

_____
Employee signature

_____
Observer signature

Name: _____   Date: _____

Skill: **Vaginal Irrigation**

Steps	Completed	Comments
1. Explain the reason and procedure to the resident.		
2. Wash your hands.		
3. Bring the supplies needed to the bedside and screen the resident.		
4. Assist the resident to use the bedpan or commode to void.		
5. Place the resident on the bedpan in the dorsal recumbent position.		
6. Drape the resident with a bath blanket for modesty, exposing only the area where you are working.		
7. Clamp the irrigation tubing and fill bag with the prescribed solution. Unclamp tubing, expel air, and reclamp the setup.		
8. Put on your gloves.		
9. Separate the labia and cleanse with gentle backward motions.		
10. Insert the nozzle backward and downward 2 to 3 inches into vagina. Hold the bag approximately 12 inches high or hang on an IV pole. Rotate the nozzle while the solution flows in.		
11. Clamp the tubing when the solution has been used. Remove the nozzle when the irrigation solution is finished and assist the resident into a sitting position to facilitate drainage. Observe the return flow.		
12. Assist the resident in drying the perineum. Wipe from front to back. Apply a perineal pad, if needed.		
13. Remove your gloves.		
13. Position resident comfortably with call light and needed personal items within reach.		
14. Wash your hands.		

Self-assessment	Evaluation/ validation methods	Levels	Type of validation	Comments
❏ Experienced ❏ Need practice ❏ Never done ❏ Not applicable (based on scope of practice)	❏ Verbal ❏ Demonstration/ observation ❏ Practical exercise ❏ Interactive class	❏ Beginner ❏ Intermediate ❏ Expert	❏ Orientation ❏ Annual ❏ Other _____	

_____
Employee signature

_____
Observer signature

© 2009 HCPro, Inc.

| Name: _____ | Date: _____ |

Skill: **Caring for the Wandering Resident**

Steps	Completed	Comments
1. Always explain the reasons and procedures to the resident.		
2. Plan care to: • Prevent a deterioration of the resident's symptoms • Preserve the resident's dignity • Promote health and the highest level independent functioning possible • Provide safety within the facility • Prevent the resident from eloping • Identify, decrease, or eliminate stressors that trigger wandering • Provide structure, repetition, consistency, and predictability in the environment • Develop a therapeutic relationship with the resident • Preserve family support and unity as much as possible		
3. Continuously reorient the resident to their own room and belongings. Provide a bedside stand, box, or other receptacle with items the resident can rummage through in the hallway, such as junk mail, old clothes, magazines, etc.		
4. Encourage group activities and attempt to keep occupied.		
5. Eliminate or decrease clutter, noise, and confusion in the environment.		
6. Ask the resident to fold towels and washcloths, or sort other harmless items.		
7. Provide a radio with a headset. Play soft, soothing music, or the resident's favorite type of music, if known; this approach is often effective when others fail.		
8. Monitor the resident's location with visual checks at least every 15 to 30 minutes. Document "verified location of resident at _____" on a flow sheet.		
9. Know and record what the resident is wearing on the assignment sheet.		

10. Put familiar items in resident's room to assist in identification.		
11. Monitor the appetite and eating, as the wandering resident has the tendency to forget to eat.		

Self-assessment	Evaluation/ validation methods	Levels	Type of validation	Comments
❏ Experienced ❏ Need practice ❏ Never done ❏ Not applicable (based on scope of practice)	❏ Verbal ❏ Demonstration/ observation ❏ Practical exercise ❏ Interactive class	❏ Beginner ❏ Intermediate ❏ Expert	❏ Orientation ❏ Annual ❏ Other _____	

_____
Employee signature

_____
Observer signature

Name: _____ Date: _____

Skill: **Weights**

Steps	Completed	Comments
1. Explain the reason and procedure to the resident. Ensure the resident's bladder is empty. If he or she is wearing an incontinent brief, change it prior to weighing the resident.		
2. Ensure that the scale is balanced on "0."		
3. Assist the resident onto the scale.		
4. Ensure that the resident is safe prior to allowing him or her to be alone on the scale.		
5. Record the weight.		
6. When using a wheelchair scale, deduct the weight of the empty wheelchair prior to recording the weight.		
7. Report fluctuations promptly to the charge nurse: • Charge nurses are to notify the physician of weight losses or gains of plus or minus 5 pounds or 5% • The dietician is to evaluate all weight losses or gains of plus or minus 5 pounds or 5% • All residents will be weighed at least monthly and upon admission		

Self-assessment	Evaluation/ validation methods	Levels	Type of validation	Comments
❏ Experienced ❏ Need practice ❏ Never done ❏ Not applicable (based on scope of practice)	❏ Verbal ❏ Demonstration/ observation ❏ Practical exercise ❏ Interactive class	❏ Beginner ❏ Intermediate ❏ Expert	❏ Orientation ❏ Annual ❏ Other _____	

_____
Employee signature

_____
Observer signature

 Competency Management in Long-Term Care

Name: _____ Date: _____

Skill: **Assessing the Carotid Artery for a Bruit**

Steps	Completed	Comments
1. Gently locate the artery on one side of the neck.		
2. Palpate the artery. Determine whether a thrill or slight vibration is present.		
3. Place the stethoscope over the carotid artery, beginning at the jaw line.		
4. Ask the resident to hold his or her breath.		
5. Lightly press the diaphragm. Auscultate while moving down the length of the artery to the clavicle.		
6. Repeat on the other side.		
7. If you feel vibration or hear a swishing sound, this suggests vessel narrowing.		
8. Inform the physician of your findings, and take other appropriate nursing action.		
9. Document your findings.		

Self-assessment	Evaluation/ validation methods	Levels	Type of validation	Comments
❏ Experienced ❏ Need practice ❏ Never done ❏ Not applicable (based on scope of practice)	❏ Verbal ❏ Demonstration/ observation ❏ Practical exercise ❏ Interactive class	❏ Beginner ❏ Intermediate ❏ Expert	❏ Orientation ❏ Annual ❏ Other _____	

_____
Employee signature

_____
Observer signature

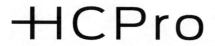